The Essentia

Energy Healing

by Dr. Michael Andron and Ben Andron

Illustrations by Rosanne Gibel

ALPHA

A member of Penguin Group (USA) Inc.

ALPHA BOOKS

Published by Penguin Group (USA) Inc.

Penguin Group (USA) Inc., 375 Hudson Street, New York, New York 10014, USA • Penguin Group (Canada), 90 Eglinton Avenue East, Suite 700, Toronto, Ontario M4P 2Y3, Canada (a division of Pearson Penguin Canada Inc.) • Penguin Books Ltd., 80 Strand, London WC2R 0RL, England • Penguin Ireland, 25 St. Stephen's Green, Dublin 2, Ireland (a division of Penguin Books Ltd.) • Penguin Group (Australia), 250 Camberwell Road, Camberwell, Victoria 3124, Australia (a division of Pearson Australia Group Pty. Ltd.) • Penguin Books India Pvt. Ltd., 11 Community Centre, Panchsheel Park, New Delhi—110 017, India • Penguin Group (NZ), 67 Apollo Drive, Rosedale, North Shore, Auckland 1311, New Zealand (a division of Pearson New Zealand Ltd.) • Penguin Books (South Africa) (Pty.) Ltd., 24 Sturdee Avenue, Rosebank, Johannesburg 2196, South Africa

Penguin Books Ltd., Registered Offices: 80 Strand, London WC2R 0RL, England

International Standard Book Number: 978-1-61564-190-1
Library of Congress Catalog Card Number: 2012930863

14   13   12   8   7   6   5   4   3   2   1

Interpretation of the printing code: The rightmost number of the first series of numbers is the year of the book's printing; the rightmost number of the second series of numbers is the number of the book's printing. For example, a printing code of 12-1 shows that the first printing occurred in 2012.

Printed in the United States of America

Note: This publication contains the opinions and ideas of its authors. It is intended to provide helpful and informative material on the subject matter covered. It is sold with the understanding that the authors and publisher are not engaged in rendering professional services in the book. If the reader requires personal assistance or advice, a competent professional should be consulted.

The authors and publisher specifically disclaim any responsibility for any liability, loss, or risk, personal or otherwise, which is incurred as a consequence, directly or indirectly, of the use and application of any of the contents of this book.

Most Alpha books are available at special quantity discounts for bulk purchases for sales promotions, premiums, fund-raising, or educational use. Special books, or book excerpts, can also be created to fit specific needs.

For details, write: Special Markets, Alpha Books, 375 Hudson Street, New York, NY 10014.

Publisher: *Marie Butler-Knight*
Associate Publisher: *Mike Sanders*
Executive Managing Editor: *Billy Fields*
Executive Acquisitions Editor: *Lori Cates Hand*
Development Editor: *Mark Reddin*
Senior Production Editor: *Janette Lynn*

Copy Editor: *Jan Zoya*
Cover Designer: *Rebecca Batchelor*
Book Designers: *Rebecca Batchelor, William Thomas*
Indexer: *Julie Bess*
Layout: *Ayanna Lacey*
Senior Proofreader: *Laura Caddell*

Dedication

I dedicate this book to two people:

To my incredible son, Ben:

For so many years in theatre, yoga, martial arts, and energy work, he was also my student. Working on this book together has been an amazing opportunity to get to know him in a whole new way as an adult and to be on the receiving end of his wisdom, understanding, and artistry.

To my remarkable wife, Lillian:

Her patience and perseverance as soul-mate, student, teacher, actor, mother, and grandmother have always been inspiring, supportive, and joyful. Without her, you'd never be reading this book. She provided the time and energy to make it all happen.

—Michael Andron

For my children, Sarah, Joseph, Elchanan, and Jacob, who are a constant inspiration, and have taught me more than they will ever realize. For my amazing wife, Michelle, who never stops pushing me to be better than what I am.

—Ben Andron

Contents

Part 3   Healing Others Starts with Healing Yourself   155

Appendixes

Introduction

Throughout history, there have been energy healers: individuals with the ability to help the sick eliminate disease or jump-start a self-healing mechanism to help them on the road to health and wellness.

In time, many of these naturally gifted healers organized their techniques into whole systems of natural healing. These systems were as diverse as the individuals and cultures that spawned them, but they all agreed on one thing: energy healing was all made possible through some kind of nonphysical medium. The healer was somehow able to tap into an unseen energy source and channel a healing message to another person.

Different cultures tried to explain these "healings" in many ways. As different philosophies and religions developed, their early practitioners provided maps as to how the world was set up and how healing could fit into their paradigm or worldview. With these maps, these systems evolved into very thorough programs for health and wellness.

Of course, the actual language and models vary according to the particular culture, but if you looked at the essence of the models side by side, you'd see that there are amazing similarities from one to the other, almost as if they're all using different words and images to describe the same phenomena.

In some cultures, these individuals and systems faded into the background as science developed a greater understanding of how the body works. Yet in other cultures, the ancient and modern systems still work side by side in a complementary fashion.

Today, science has evolved to the point where some of the ancient attempts to explain these phenomena might be better understood and more freely utilized, if we could just open our minds to the possibilities.

The first thing to realize is that the word "energy" is not a metaphor. The energy that facilitates healing is real, even if we don't fully understand it yet. I'll present a working hypothesis in this book. While it's certainly not the final word on how it works or the "science behind it all," keep in mind that the word "science" comes from a Latin root meaning "to know." We're just at the beginning of understanding that knowledge about energy healing, a phenomenon that has worked for centuries.

You, the Reader

Some of you may be new to the subject of energy healing, and this stuff might be a little foreign to you. Please know there is nothing wrong with being skeptical—as long as you are an open-minded skeptic. When you watch a movie, for example, you have to suspend your disbelief. You ignore the fact that some of what you're watching doesn't exist in our day-to-day reality, but you go along with it to get the essence of the story. In the case of energy healing, just because some of this can't be fully explained with modern science (yet), come along for the ride and see what happens!

If you have experience with a particular modality of energy healing, you may have an easier time with some of the broader concepts in this book. I would ask you, however, to suspend your disbelief as well. It's difficult to look at all the different systems and not get caught up in which one is better, or right, or how this explanation isn't exactly the way your teacher taught you—it's perfectly normal and happens to everyone.

When I think of how an exploration of energy healing should be, I picture a mountaintop, where all the masters and originators of major religions, philosophies, and systems of meditation and healing are all happily sipping tea and discussing with each other how wondrous it is that there are so many diverse ways of perfecting the world. A garden of so many different colors of flowers, if you will! The dark side of this vision is down at the base of the mountain, where all of their followers are fighting, arguing, and even killing each other over whose system is right, and best, and why all the others are wrong, or not as advanced as theirs is.

Let's all try to explore the world of energy healing together, from the top of that mountain.

My Personal Background

Because we'll be spending some time together, let me introduce myself. Beginning in 1963, I spent several decades in pretty intense training in yoga, martial arts, and natural healing. These diverse arts are linked by a common theme: they're all about using energy for personal and global healing. I was fortunate enough to spend many years with some most remarkable teachers. Because you'll be hearing some of their ideas, lessons, and stories throughout the book, let me introduce them now.

Greta Woodrew, my late sister, was my first teacher in healing. She taught me to be *in* the world, but not *of* it. Keep your roots grounded in the academic study of energy healing, but don't let it prevent you from dreaming and reaching upward toward a higher light.

My yoga teacher was Madame Blanche DeVries, a pioneer teacher of yoga in the West. Beyond the postures and breathing, she maintained that the first, and last, lesson in yoga is character, and advocated moderation in all things.

Prof. Harvey Sober, my martial arts Grand Master of internal and external martial arts, has energy control that is legendary. Healing, he teaches, is an essential part of authentic martial arts training. It's not enough to take a man apart; you have to be able to put him back together!

The late Dr. Andrija Puharich, MD, was a neurologist, published author, and medical researcher with over 80 patents in medical technology to his credit. His understanding of energy healing and his insights into the physics of healing have guided me for decades.

My hope in this book is to share with you a perspective that comes from over four decades of these studies, and to challenge you with some life-changing ideas and stories.

How to Use This Book

In *The Essential Guide to Energy Healing*, we'll look at the history, science, and scope of energy healing. I'll share actual cases, and prepare you to ask the right questions about energy healing. I hope that as an opened-minded seeker of truth, you'll try to understand, appreciate, and learn from the exploration.

In **Part 1, Understanding the Theories and Methods of Energy Healing,** we'll establish a common vocabulary and working paradigm that we can use throughout the book to survey a broad variety of approaches to energy healing, as they come from many diverse cultures, worldviews, and languages. We'll look at ancient systems and modern science, to discover views that are remarkably similar. We'll also look at how energy healing deals with managing stress, the single-greatest threat to our lives today. Finally, we'll "get real" by answering questions that so many people have when first entering the world of energy healing.

Part 2, Energy Healing Systems, surveys a sampling of the many systems of energy healing. Though it's beyond the scope of this guide to cover every single healing system, we'll deal with approaches to energy diagnosis, laying on of hands, massage, and healing with needles, crystals, water, homeopathic remedies, electricity, and many others. We'll also look at remote healing, or healing done from a distance.

In **Part 3, Healing Others Starts with Healing Yourself,** we'll learn some basic skills that will enhance your energy healing experience, either as a healer or a patient. We'll cover the basics of breathing, centering, ocular divergence, and self-massage. To help in this training, you'll be able to access short instructional videos, as it's easier to learn some of these skills if you see them.

Finally, in **Part 4, Lessons from the World of Energy Healing,** we'll help you figure out what kind of healer you want to see, or what kind of healer you want to be, by focusing on some questions you might ask a healer, as well as the questions you should be asking yourself. I'll also share some personal case-studies and experiences that had interesting lessons to teach.

Essential Extras

Throughout the book we'll try to "spice up the salad" by clarifying the information in the text with sidebars that will help you along:

Unless you've studied energy healing and science extensively, you'll encounter unfamiliar terminology in this book. These definition sidebars will help.

Deeper connections

Background facts, supporting information, and additional insights in these sidebars will ease your exploration of the world of energy healing.

stay Grounded These sidebars will alert you to common misconceptions, potential problem areas, and some of the traps that students encounter. Pay careful attention!

You'll also see a fourth, name-changing sidebar that presents anecdotes, interesting facts, case histories, or other extended background information you should know.

Acknowledgments

From Michael Andron:

In addition to Ben's incredible list of accomplishments as writer, producer, playwright, and martial artist, he has shown himself to be a master at choosing Michelle, the most wonderful mate imaginable. Her generosity of time has supported this book immeasurably. Together, they have drawn four old souls into this world to be our grandchildren. What more could a father ask for?

I have to bow to my teachers, on whose shoulders one always stands, in the order they shared their light with me:

> I thank my late sister Greta Woodrew, whom I got to know best as teacher in yoga and healing (we were born over 20 years apart), who got me started in all this. It was the exact 1-year anniversary of her "graduation" that the agreement on this book was confirmed. Thanks, Gret!

> I thank Prof. H. I. Sober, my life-long master teacher in martial arts, energy, and life lessons. Like a father teaching his child to walk, he knew just how many steps back to take, and how slowly to take them, to keep me moving forward.

> I thank Madame Blanche DeVries, pioneer teacher of yoga in the West, who took a young man in his early 20's and guided him for a decade in the technique and character lessons of yoga.

I thank Dr. Andrija Puharich, whose knowledge, encouragement, and sense of humor were always inspiring.

It's true; you learn almost as much from your students, especially when they reach their own levels of mastery. They continue to be friends and colleagues and bring great light to the world. All have helped in the creation of this *Essential Guide.*

I thank Jack and Dr. Amanda Heinemann, students in martial arts and energy healing, and two of the most selfless, supportive friends one could hope for. They heard each chapter in early drafts, and helped in any way they could!

I thank Andrew Chernick, DAc, who took each wild idea in yoga, martial arts, and energy healing to heart and to fruition and has never lost his focus.

I thank Harvey Grossbard, OMD, who began yoga and healing with me as a teen 35 years ago and has never stopped growing. His contributions to this work are significant.

In acknowledging both teachers and students, I must extend my deepest love and gratitude to the one person that has been both for me for over 40 years, my wife Lillian. All of this is thanks to her devotion and love. I know she'd rather I didn't write these words for her … but how can I not? In addition to being the embodiment of the kind radiant energy we talk about throughout this book, she is also a master of martial arts and a yoga adept, and has taught by my side and has been at my side for over four decades.

I cannot thank Rosanne Gibel enough for her amazing illustrations that contribute so much to this book, as well as for her friendship and collaboration in our theatre-work over decades.

I gratefully thank Aaron Zippin for his generosity, expertise, and caring in producing the series of short videos that will serve as a complement to this book and make the learning a lot easier for the reader.

I thank Jonathan Yunger, a forever-kind-of-student in theatre and energy healing, who, without knowing it at the time, planted the synchronistic seed for this book.

I offer much thanks to Bart Ostroff, MA, CMH, my guide in hypnosis, for his helpful contributions, and always inspiring and fun emails.

To my dear friends who read the early manuscripts and provided critique, insights, and motivation: Yoram Padeh, MD, and Andee Chonin, EdD, RN.

To my agent and now friend, Rita Battat Silverman, and Leap Over It, Inc., who sought me out for this adventure, and whose enthusiasm and optimism have kept us going throughout the rapid, yet arduous, process of creating a book.

Thanks to Randy Landenheim-Gil, our first tier editor, for her expertise and patience. She kept us on our toes throughout.

To Mark Reddin, Lori Cates Hand, Janette Lynn, and the whole Alpha group of wizards who turned our manuscript into a beautiful and meaningful reality.

I offer love and gratitude to Hiro Emoto and Michiko Hayashi of Office Masaru Emoto for their friendship, helpfulness, and caring.

To Jenny Davis at Magic Eye, Inc. for her generosity of time, caring, and energy.

To Monica Sanchez, Reiki Master, for her helpful clarifications and discussions.

To Carolyn Kay Wheeler, RN, Program Coordinator and teacher at Pumpkin Hollow Retreat, the center of Therapeutic Touch, a student of its co-founders since 1972. You went above and beyond my questions in your review and clarification.

From Ben Andron:

When my father was exploring the nature of the universe in Dr. Puharich's lab, I was playing in the river that ran through his front yard. My first time in a martial arts dojo was when I was 13 days old. I tumbled on DeVries's yoga mat as a baby. I've visited ashrams, met swamis, meditated in the Great Pyramid—and that was all before Junior High.

Growing up under that influence instilled in me a deep spiritual awareness that has guided me throughout my life. My father was my first teacher in the martial arts, meditation, yoga, theatre—and his guidance has contributed to everything I do. Working on this book together with him was an opportunity to reestablish my connection to the beautiful world of energy healing. I am so grateful for the privilege of helping him to share his knowledge and wisdom with the world, and for sharing it with me throughout my life.

My mother has been a constant pillar of support and encouragement in everything I do. I would like to thank her for that, and also hanging in there during this long and difficult process.

I would like to thank my wife, Michelle, who went to bed alone on too many occasions because we were working late on this book. Her constant support made this possible.

I would like to thank my children Sarah, Joseph, Elchanan, and Jacob for bringing joy and significance to every day.

During my childhood, Master Sober was like a grandfather to me. As I grew up, he also became my master. I would like to thank him for his teaching, guidance, and encouragement. They have brought me to a level of mastery I never thought possible, and continue to push me further.

I would also like to thank Sifu Gus Rubio and Sifu Qichen Guo for opening my eyes to so many different forms of generating Qi.

I would like to thank my student and friend Darren Melameth for inspiring me on a weekly basis to develop a greater understanding of the energy all around us.

I would like to thank Mr. C. for always encouraging my writing and teaching me the eternal value of a good thesis sentence.

Lastly, I would like to thank Rita Battat Silverman, Randy Ladenheim-Gil, Mark Reddin, Lori Cates Hand, and everyone at Alpha who made this book a reality.

Special Thanks to the Technical Reviewers

The Essential Guide to Energy Healing was reviewed by experts who double-checked the accuracy of what you'll learn here, to help us ensure that this book gives you the essentials on energy healing. Special thanks are extended to Dr. Lorna Minewiser and Yoram Padeh, MD.

Trademarks

All terms mentioned in this book that are known to be or are suspected of being trademarks or service marks have been appropriately capitalized. Alpha Books and Penguin Group (USA) Inc. cannot attest to the accuracy of this information. Use of a term in this book should not be regarded as affecting the validity of any trademark or service mark.

Part 1

Understanding the Theories and Methods of Energy Healing

Our worldview, or paradigm, is the lens through which we see, interpret, and understand everything in our lives. Because we all have different paradigms, worldviews, and experiences, the first thing we have to do is build a common vocabulary for the world of energy.

Then we'll go back in time to understand some of the early cultures that developed and utilized energy healing. How did they view the world? How did they understand energy healing as part of their worldview?

We'll also look at the world of modern science and physics to see if there is a scientific explanation for some of the more "out there" stuff that happens as a result of energy healing. We'll examine both the physical and energy components of stress, the source of many illnesses for which we might seek energy healing.

And finally, we'll bring our discussion down to Earth, and address certain questions, concerns, and reservations that keep coming up, some of which have probably already occurred to you.

chapter 1

What Is Energy Healing?

Establishing a common worldview and vocabulary

The difference between curing and healing

The trickle-down, trickle-up phenomenon

Using ancient paradigms and modern science
to better understand energy healing

To understand and fully appreciate energy healing,
we must look at it through the eyes of its practitioners
and early developers. Because many of the ancient
healing arts were developed in the East, we may need
to adjust our contemporary Western paradigm to really
understand them. We'll also need to develop a common
working vocabulary to make it easier for us to explore
and understand the varied systems.

Developing an Energy Healing Vocabulary

Before we begin exploring some individual healing
systems, I want to make sure we're all speaking the
same language. You might be wondering what I mean
when I say energy. "Do you mean Qi (pronounced *Chi*),
Ki, Reiki, Prana, Manna, Ru'aō, Orgone, Ohr Āyn Sōf,
bioplasmic energy, hado, 'the force,' ether, or something
else?" The answer is "Yes." I'm actually talking about *all*
of them.

There is one universal energy that exists on many frequencies and goes by many names. Ever since the biblical story of the Tower of Babel, when everyone began speaking different languages, words have been a problem.

It seems there have always been psychics, prophets, and mystic seers in the world. These special individuals could tune in to a different reality, sensing something no one else around them could. Each would enter an *altered state of consciousness* and see or hear or experience something.

Finding Meaning

Altered states of consciousness refer to brain wave patterns. The normal waking brain wave is 15–30 cycles per second or hertz (hz), beta. When you relax, go to sleep, or just slow down, you enter alpha, 8–14 hz. Deep relaxation or deep trance is theta, 4–7 hz; the sleep state is delta, 1–3 hz. The best frequency for healing is deep alpha or high theta, around 8 hz.

When they came back to normal consciousness, they tried to communicate what they received. Some wrote poetry. Some drew pictures. Some composed music. Of course, each one of them came from a different culture and spoke a different language, but if you compare what they saw— and we will—you'll begin to see striking similarities.

Let's start with something big … like the universe! Scientists tell us that 95 percent of the universe is hydrogen. Even in the vacuum of outer space, you'll find a hydrogen atom every cubic centimeter. If your eyes were super-microscopes, you could see that those atoms actually are made up of smaller particles (protons, electrons, etc.) and that those particles are made up of even smaller particles (quarks, monopoles, strings, etc.). If you could go smaller still, you'd discover that these super tiny particles aren't particles at all. They're energy flux. The entire universe, if you could see to the smallest level possible, is an infinite ocean of energy. In this instance, at least, physics and metaphysics agree.

In this book I'll call this ocean of energy the WEB, a worldwide energy bubble. Everything we know to exist in the universe is inside that bubble, as well as all the things we suspect but don't know for certain. This particular model is based on an ancient *Kabbalistic* view. I'll present a simplified explanation of that model in the next chapter.

The word Kabbalah comes from a Hebrew word meaning "to receive." **Kabbalistic** studies were intended for those who were learned in Jewish tradition and practice as a way to provide deeper insight and understanding of the Torah, the Jewish bible, Talmud, and Jewish practice. It provides deep meditative teaching about the WEB.

You've probably never heard the term WEB, or worldwide energy bubble, used when referring to energy. I've found that using more general terms often helps us get past the different words and understand the concept in a more universal way. We'll be using a number of computer metaphors throughout the course of this book, which will hopefully make our study more accessible. In this case, the WEB will refer to the myriad of terms out there for this universal energy ocean.

So if this WEB is an ocean filled with all the energy (and matter, too, which is just dense energy) in the universe, wouldn't it be great to learn how to access it? How can we do that?

Let's come back down to earth and look at our own bodies. Your body is made up of bones, tissue, fluid, etc., all of which are made up of cells. Cells are made up of molecules and molecules are made up of atoms. And atoms, as we mentioned, are themselves made up of flux: pure energy. Actually, as science might see us, we're each a field or a matrix of energy that serves as a kind of energy mold into which our body fits. If your eyes could see what's really there, we'd all look like the shimmering lights when someone beams up on *Star Trek*. Everything made up of matter is, at its core, really just energy flux. That leads us to our next key vocabulary word: I call the body's field the energy matrix.

Each and every one of you is an energy matrix existing inside the WEB. And here's the key: your energy matrix and the WEB are both made of the same stuff. That means you can use your energy matrix to log on to the WEB.

Think of your energy matrix as a ladder. In the book of Genesis, Jacob dreams of a ladder rooted to the earth, with its top reaching the heavens. There are angels going up and down the ladder. And Jacob realizes that God is in this "place." The place is the WEB, and the ladder—the way we can climb up and down—is our energy matrix, connecting the universe's higher energies to our individual lower energies. Or, if you're so inclined, connecting heaven and earth.

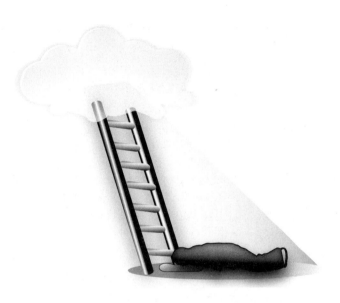

An illustration of Jacob's ladder.

Dreaming Big

The beauty of Jacob's dream is in a little-noticed fact: the angels are go-ing up and down the ladder. Don't angels live in heaven? Shouldn't they come down before they go up? The answer lies in the Hebrew word for angel, *mal'ach*, which means both angel and messenger. We humans are at the base of the ladder. We send our messenger-angels up the ladder and, in biblical terms, the Creator reaches back down to us.

So our energy matrix is the energy component of our bodies, and it functions like a ladder that enables us to reach higher levels of the WEB.

Why aren't you already using your energy matrix to access the WEB? The truth is, you are, at least on a very basic level. It's not just the light and heat of the sun that sustains your life on Earth. The very life force that flows through you and keeps you alive comes from the WEB. Just by being alive, you're accessing one of the more basic frequencies of energy from the WEB.

But the WEB has higher, faster frequencies of energy within it, too. In order for you to tune into those higher frequencies, you need security clearance, so to speak. You have to upgrade your energy matrix.

Let's use a radio analogy to explain further. Radio stations are broadcasting at many different frequencies, but they can't all be accessed on the same receiver. If you only have an AM radio, you won't be able to tune in to FM, Satellite Radio, Short Wave radio frequencies, and so on.

The WEB is broadcasting on many frequencies, also. If you have a highly developed energy matrix, you can receive higher level frequencies from the WEB. If not, you'll just get the basic life-sustaining energies you need.

Energy healers utilize their energy matrixes to log on to higher and higher frequencies of healing energy from the WEB. A healer with a more developed energy matrix will be able to access higher healing energies and be more successful with his or her healing.

One last vocabulary clarification: Throughout the book, when I use the words patient, diagnose, or treat, I'm always using them in the context of energy healing and not conventional medicine, unless otherwise indicated.

The Paradigm for Energy Healing

In simple terms, a paradigm is a worldview. A more textbook definition is that it's a set of rules, ideas, and principles that govern and define everything on a particular subject.

Let's take a quick look at the paradigm of Newtonian physics. If you have one of those problems we all hated in school—two trains, X kilometers apart, are on a collision course, traveling at a velocity of such-and-such, will decelerate at a rate of Y—the Newtonian paradigm gives us the tools you need to solve it, if you can remember high school physics.

But what happens when something comes along that doesn't fit within the parameters of the paradigm? The paradigm will either try to make it fit or will ignore it completely. While most problems about how things work in our visible world are answered by the rules of Newtonian physics, questions about things that are very much smaller and very much larger are not. Sub-atomic particles, for example, require a broader paradigm to solve their riddles. So do galactic-size dilemmas. These kinds of problems require a different, broader set of rules and principles: *quantum physics*. What scientists call *Newtonian-Cartesian physics* is a special case within the larger paradigm of quantum physics. It's not that Newton and Descartes were wrong; it's that their paradigms were limited to defining only what was within their boundaries.

Finding Meaning

Quantum physics, developed in the early twentieth century, tries to explain the behavior of the very small and very large aspects of matter and energy. **Newtonian-Cartesian physics,** also known as Newtonian or classical physics, deals with the physical world of the senses: what we can see, hear, smell, taste, and touch. Energy healing is best studied and understood within the paradigm of quantum physics.

One doesn't have to go to such extremes to see paradigms at work. Pasteur's discoveries of the little bugs called germs that caused disease didn't fit into the medical paradigm of his day. And what about computers in every home and cell phones for every child? Our parents could never have imagined such a thing when they were growing up.

When I was growing up, you never heard about acupuncture on TV. It didn't fit into the Western model of medicine until the 1970s and is still rejected by some physicians. Today, however, you can tune in to medical shows in prime time and see storylines involving acupuncture and homeopathy.

Slowly the medical paradigm is expanding and shifting. It's opening up and reaching new territories within its boundaries. Energy, although not as we are discussing it in this book, is a common term in Western medicine in the form of X-rays, CAT scans, MRIs, ultrasound, and laser surgery. We have entered an era where waves are as much a part of medicine as were setting bones and cutting people open 100 years ago. The same way that Newtonian physics became a special case within the larger paradigm of quantum physics, you could argue that Newtonian medicine is becoming a special case within the larger paradigm of quantum medicine.

This development is closing the gap between conventional Western medicine and energy healing, due in large part to Doctors Larry Dossey, Deepak Chopra, Bernie Siegal, Norman Shealy, and others. Other doctors, including Andrija Puharich, Robert Becker, and other paradigm researcher-iconoclasts, laid the groundwork for the science of energy healing. It's going to take the credibility that comes with all those MD and other academic letters after their names for their work to enter the mainstream. The current medical establishment will rarely allow an acupuncturist, hypno-therapist, or healer to change anything, even if they're achieving amazing clinical results.

Iconoclasts Pave the Way

An iconoclast is an idol smasher, someone who tries to break up out-dated ideas and dogmas that he or she believes are no longer valid, and to build new visions of the world. One of the early iconoclasts was the biblical Abraham who, as legend has it, smashed the idols in his father's shop and then told his father the idols had smashed themselves. When his father said that was impossible—they were just statues!—Abraham replied, "So, if they are powerless, why do you bow down to them?" Dad got the message.

A clear knowledge of one's own paradigm is important in energy healing. If a patient I'm working with is operating within a different paradigm, my words of comfort or instruction may elicit confusion, anger, even fear, simply because the vocabulary I use may mean something different to me than it does to him.

The Difference Between Curing and Healing

Whenever I give a lecture, or work with a patient, I hear a lot of the same questions over and over again. Here's one question I've answered hundreds of times over the years: what's the difference between curing and healing?

When I use the term curing, I'm referring to the elimination of a disease or the symptoms of a disease. Sometimes the cure is simple. You stub your toe, you have pain, and your doctor treats it. Because he knows the cause of the pain, he may give you something to take for personal comfort. The bone heals, the pain stops, and you stop taking the aspirin. Simple.

But sometimes it's not so clear-cut. Pain can be a signal to let you know that something is wrong somewhere else in the body: a referred pain. Let's say you have a kidney stone. There are no sensory nerves in your ureter (the tube that connects the bladder to the kidney where kidney stones often get stuck), so you can't feel the stone. Your ureter, which is connected to your autonomic nervous system, sends a message to your peripheral nervous system that, in turn, gives you a pain anywhere from your back/flank to your groin (or everything in between) to get your attention. Now that's a message you can feel! You go to the doctor, she does some tests and discovers your kidney stone; she does whatever procedure is necessary to get it to go away (surgery, ultra-sound, medications, etc.). Then the referred pain in your back disappears. The cause of your symptom has been discovered, treated, and you are cured.

Now, when I use the term healing—specifically energy healing—as opposed to curing, I refer to helping someone be more whole. It definitely involves trying to find the cause of the problem and not just making the symptoms go away, but it's not limited to physical causes.

To continue with our kidney stone analogy, we need to find out what took place inside your body to begin with that caused the formation of that stone, be it physical, emotional, or even spiritual. That stone could be a sign of some deeper problem. Acupuncturists will try to determine whether you have excessive fear in your life. I know what you're thinking: "Fear?! But we're talking about kidneys!" Exactly. Kidney issues, within the paradigm of energy healing, are often related to fear.

If all this talk of organs, emotions, and their inter-connections has you worried that every little symptom might be a major health breakdown, relax! These are energy connections, and they often balance themselves out without your having to do anything. Don't forget, your physical body also has bacteria and other germs that it fights off naturally. The energy matrix does the same thing to many energy imbalances.

Sometimes, healing can help the patient become more whole even when the disease, unfortunately, can't be cured. With a terminal illness, a patient may need some time to gain a deeper perspective on life—or on death. Helping a patient die with a sense of wholeness is also a gift of healing, though obviously not a cure. But our primary objective is to both heal and cure; helping a patient find her wholeness and making the disease go away.

As Above, So Below; As Below, So Above

Sometimes physical ailments affect the energy body, and sometimes energy imbalances affect the physical body.

In the case of the kidney stone, we might think of the physical disease (the cause) sending a horizontal message. That is, the body is sending a message through to a different part of the body. It's all in the body; it's all on the same frequency. It's horizontal.

Sometimes, however, the message is a vertical one. A doctor of Chinese medicine looking at the same kidney stone will do what's necessary to prompt the body to heal itself (energy massage, needles, herbs, etc.). But he'll also look at imbalances higher up within the energy matrix. This doctor knows, based on what the Chinese call the five-element theory (more on that in Chapter 2), that the emotion of fear is related to the kidneys, so he'll explore the psycho-emotional or deeper spiritual imbalance of the patient as well as the disease. If it started as an emotional imbalance, the energy problem can trickle down (vertically) within your energy matrix and send the same physical symptom (the pain) as the one that came from the horizontal source.

It can also go the other way. When you break a bone, aside from everything the physical body does to heal itself, the injury also creates an energy red alert. The physical break sends you a message of pain so you'll be careful while the bone is healing. Soon, the bone heals. But the energy scar might actually remain, perhaps because of the muscle tension you developed during the healing process. The physical injury trickled up the energy matrix and left that energy scar.

But it might not end there. The energy scar might send you a trickle-down pain for years after the bone has healed. Because the source is higher up on the energy matrix, the medical doctors you consult might not find a physical cause for your ongoing pain. They might send you to a psychologist, who can't find any neurosis causing the pain, either. An energy healer, though, might discover the energy scar: she can remove it—like removing plaque from a hard-to-reach place in your mouth—and balance the energy matrix. Now the old, outdated pain will go away.

Keeping a Balanced Mind

So far in this chapter I've introduced a Kabbalistic model to define the WEB, Chinese medicine to explain how the energy matrix can send referred message-symptoms to the body, and an example from quantum physics to better describe the energy matrix and the WEB.

This might give you the impression that you have to be an expert in all sorts of things to understand energy healing. You don't. You can participate in energy healing without any of that foundation and, hopefully, have a wonderful result.

But I look at it this way: because we were created with a left hemisphere of the brain to deal with cognitive issues and a right hemisphere to deal with more artistic, creative, and spiritual issues beyond the left brain's logic, then we should use both hemispheres when studying a subject. I want to benefit from energy healing and receive its results, but I also want to understand it to the best of my ability. I can listen to a great singer and enjoy the experience, but if I know the intricacies of voice control, pitch, and vibrato, I can enjoy the performance even more.

The Sounds of Change

When I was a kid I loved watching Louis Armstrong, the famous trumpeter, perform on TV. He had a certain magnetic energy about him—there's that word again! In celebration of the hundredth anniversary of his birth a few years ago, a program on NPR explained some of the things he did that no other musician had ever done before. I had no idea what an innovator he was in the development of jazz and blues. Since then, I appreciate his music all the more.

So even if all the background material isn't your thing, I suggest you do your best to read through the next couple of chapters without worry. In the long run, I believe you'll appreciate what follows all the more.

Essential Takeaways

- Energy healing has been around for millennia but has been described using many different words and visual models.
- You are an energy matrix living in an ocean of energy that's all around us (a worldwide energy bubble, or WEB).
- Your energy matrix has the ability to log on to the WEB and download healing energy and wisdom from it.

- Curing means having a symptom or disease go away, without necessarily addressing a deeper cause of imbalance. Healing means making someone more whole, centered, in control of his or her total holistic destiny.

- A problem in the body can trickle up to the energy matrix or trickle down to the physical body, manifesting as a symptom or disease.

- The best solution to a health issue is to address the physical problem with medical science when you can, and also address the imbalance in the energy matrix.

chapter 2

Ancient Approaches to Energy Healing

Introducing the body's energy anatomy

The basics of yoga healing

The basics of t'ai chi healing

The basics of Kabbalah's paradigm

What these approaches have in common
with our energy paradigm

In the last chapter, you saw that there are many different names for energy that come from different cultures and energy healing systems. But despite the different words, there's only one design for what we're calling the energy matrix, and one WEB (worldwide energy bubble). Therefore, we need to look at the anatomy of the energy matrix and the WEB to see the commonality between the different systems and clarify how they work.

The Body's Energy Anatomy

The human body is an amazing machine. Its many different systems all operate harmoniously to keep us alive and functioning. On the frame of the musculoskeletal system there are many other systems: circulatory (including blood and lymph), glandular, neurological, respiratory, defense-immune, reproductive, genitourinary, digestive, and more. And every one of these systems is divided into even more sub-categories, each with their own trained specialists. I knew someone who had to have a cyst removed from her eyelid. She went to the office of two eye surgeons who only did eyelids. And, more amazingly, each of the doctors specialized in either the upper or lower lid. True story!

With so many different specialties in the medical world, it's only logical that there are different systems of energy healing as well. But while yoga healing seems to deal with chakras, prana, and kundalini (terms used in yoga that I'll explain shortly) and t'ai chi healing deals with meridians and qi, there is only one energy matrix, one WEB, and one energy. These methods of healing are all related to each other in some way.

It's absurd, of course, to think that only the Chinese have meridians and only the Hindus and Buddhists have chakras. The different systems evolved because the originators, millennia ago, encountered the energy matrix in their own way and discovered how to interact with and heal it.

> **Deeper connections**
>
> The different names and systems of energy healing remind me of the well-known story of the blind men and the elephant. Each blind man was told to touch an elephant and describe what it looked like. The first man touched the ear and described the elephant as a flat, floppy, somewhat leathery creature. The one who touched the tusk described a long, smooth, hard object with a point at one end. The one who touched the leg said an elephant was like a tree, strong, vertical, and rough on the outside. You get the point.

Let's take a look at some of the systems. The purpose here is to focus on the big picture of energy healing, and how these systems are each talking about the same basic ideas using different words and different emphasis. Looking closely at these three systems should not be misconstrued as dismissing the validity and importance of the myriad of others; these three simply provide the clearest examples of how many of these systems, while seemingly very different, are at their core quite similar.

To really understand the nuances of any individual system could take a lifetime of study, so we're just going to give a broad overview of what you need to know about these systems specifically for energy healing.

Yoga Healing

You might think of yoga as the stretching class at your local gym, but yoga healing is actually one of the most widely practiced systems of energy healing. Native to India, yoga literally means union and refers to the union of body, energy, and spirit. Yoga healing is a general term alluding to the many different healing aspects in yoga.

All of the various forms of yoga—and there are a lot of them—have the same goal: perfecting what we're calling our energy matrix through character development, exercise, breathing, meditation, study, and service, enabling us to log on to the WEB and download the wisdom and healing energies that exist there. Also, new approaches to yoga have developed over the years, some more extreme in nature, others more gentle; some more flowing in movement, some more static.

MISC.

Diluted for Demand

Some of the yoga classes at the gym are watered-down versions of traditional hatha yoga, which would include lessons in character, postures, and rather intense breathing practices. The same thing happened as martial arts became popular in the United States. The bigger the demand, the more diluted the systems became to fill the need.

As we've discussed, the word WEB is obviously not part of the yoga vocabulary. Practitioners of yoga would use the word Brahm, referring to the Oneness of the universe—our WEB! In the entrance to my yoga master DeVries's home there was a beautifully carved metal sculpture that stated "All, indeed, is Brahm." The saying was a perpetual reminder that everything *within* the WEB is made of that one universal, intelligent light.

In addition to this focus on one universal light, there is a tremendous focus on what we're calling the energy matrix and its specific anatomy. The word generally used for energy in yoga is prana, which can mean life force, breath, or vital energy. There are ancient pictures of the nadis, which are the energy channels that carry needed prana/energy around the energy matrix, kind of like an energy nervous system. The word "nadi" comes from the root "nad," which means motion. And if the nadis are the nerves of the energy nervous system, then the sushumna, the central energy passageway, would be the energy spine.

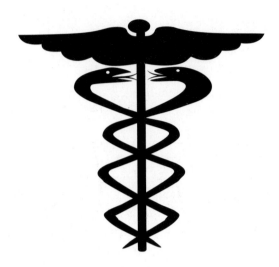

Sushumna/Caduceus.

Yoga teaches that the energy matrix has at least 72,000 nadis. When they're balanced and purified, the body will heal itself more effectively. When the student wants to "upgrade" the energy matrix for purposes of higher spiritual work, he or she will meditate on the energy nerve plexuses, the chakras, and attempt to purify them and prepare them to receive and channel a more powerful energy. This energy is known as "serpent" energy, or kundalini, and is described as coiled at the base of your spine. When it is awakened, it can rise through the chakra "plexuses" of the sushumna nadi, which, in turn, results in the yogi's higher state of consciousness.

Did You Know?

The symbol of the serpent energy awakening and rising up the center toward higher consciousness appears in two other contexts. It's the herald's staff carried by Hermes (the Roman god Mercury) and the symbol for the U.S. Army medical corps.

Let's elaborate on the chakras, since that is a term you'll encounter quite often. Chakra, the Sanskrit word for wheel, is the energy matrix's equivalent of the body's nerve plexuses and endocrine glands combined. There are seven chakras, each with a specific function in the energy matrix that parallels a function in the physical body.

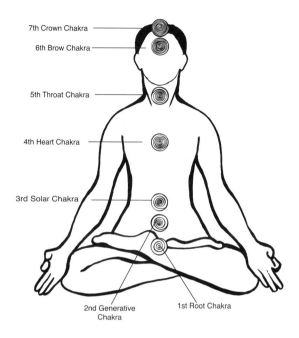

7th Crown Chakra

6th Brow Chakra

5th Throat Chakra

4th Heart Chakra

3rd Solar Chakra

2nd Generative Chakra

1st Root Chakra

The body's seven chakras.

The 7 Chakras and Their Correspondences

Chakra	Traditional Metaphors	Physical/Energy Counterpart	Physical/Energy Function
1	Physical	Uterus Prostate Rectal Plexus	Eliminations-Control, Stress Center
2	Emotional	Ovaries/Testes Inferior-Mesenteric-Plexus	Genetic Regulator, Sexual Energy Regulator
3	Intellectual	Adrenal Glands Solar Plexus	Digestive Control, Fight-or-Flight Regulator, Defense-Immune Regulator, Stress Center

continues

The 7 Chakras and Their Correspondences   continued

Chakra	Traditional Metaphors	Physical/Energy Counterpart	Physical/Energy Function
4	Empathy	Thymus Gland Cardiac Plexus	Defense-Immune Control, Negative Ion Balance, Circulatory Regulator
5	Creativity Expressivity	Thyroid Gland Medulla	Breath Control, Chemical Regulator (pH Balance), Circulation Control, Stress Center
6	Intuition	Pituitary Gland Hypothalamus	Master Hormonal Control, Metabolic Control
7	Spiritual	Pineal Gland Thalamus	Electro-Magnetic Receiver

If you've ever passed a power station, you've seen warning signs referring to high voltage. If thousands of volts came directly into your home, they would fry the electrical system and probably burn down your house. There has to be a system of transformers that steps down the voltage and delivers the power at a level your house can handle: 110v for most of the appliances, and maybe 220v for some of the heavier equipment.

Think of chakras as step-down transformers in the energy matrix. The very high energy coming down from the WEB would short-circuit your energy matrix if it wasn't first stepped down and distributed to the various systems that need it, each at a level they can handle. First, the higher chakras draw down the prana/energy from the WEB and slow it down to the speed it needs. That chakra then distributes the slowed-down energy to the right place through the nadis, or slows it down even more and passes it on to the next lower chakra.

Chakras are never asleep and don't need to be awakened. If the chakras were closed, as some teachers suggest, and it was up to *you* to open them, you would die. However, they can be upgraded to enable the energy matrix to receive a higher level of energy from the WEB. The concept of opening or awakening a chakra versus upgrading may sound like semantics, but the distinction is critical. Remember, the chakras are the step-down transformers of the body, and the energy they supply and distribute is what keeps all your physical systems running. If you're alive, the chakras are working.

One of the most common metaphors for the chakras is that each of the seven corresponds to a part of the human condition. The first chakra represents the physical, the second chakra the emotional, the third chakra the intellectual, the fourth (heart) chakra caring and loving, the fifth (throat) chakra creativity (it's near the mouth and arms, the organs of creative expression), the sixth chakra intuition, and the seventh chakra the spirit. Based on that metaphor, students who want to open their hearts to become more loving might meditate on the fourth or heart chakra.

The chakras themselves have very specific biological energy activities to keep your body running smoothly. So while you're meditating on love and caring—a metaphor but not a body function—you're also affecting the actual organs controlled by the fourth chakra: the heart, the main hydraulic pump and negative-ion generator of your body, and the thymus gland, which produces T-cells for the immune system.

stay Grounded

Meditation on chakras, if not done properly, can cause serious problems. A woman who had been meditating excessively with a well-known guru came to see me with chest pains. She was in continuous pain with no conventional medical reason for it. She had so over-meditated on her fourth chakra—approximately four hours a day—that it had short-circuited. How could meditation have caused such problems? Because energy isn't just a metaphor; it's real!

In addition to their biological relationships, each chakra also has a psycho-emotional component and, at an even higher energy level, a psycho-spiritual aspect as well. Think of each level (the physical, the emotional, and the spiritual) as octaves on a piano, and the chakras are the seven notes within each. In the first octave, the third chakra, for example, is related to fight or flight. One octave higher—on the psycho-emotional level—that same chakra (or note) is linked to the emotional ability to assert or yield appropriately to stressful events. This can be a little complicated, but the important thing to remember is that these energies contribute to how your energy matrix relates to your body, emotions, and psycho-spiritual being.

The chakras need to be worked on and developed as a continuum or the system will be out of sync with itself. You can't just pick one of them and work on that in isolation from the others. Think of them as a temple. You might be inclined to focus most of your energy on your meditation room, but if you don't also take the garbage out, the smell is going to make it really hard for you to concentrate.

The key to yoga is cleaning out the body, deepening your breathing skills, quieting your mind, and working to upgrade your energy matrix on all levels to enable you to log on to the WEB and download higher energy to share through teaching and energy healing. All this has to be worked on over time, together. Remember, yoga means union.

T'ai Chi Healing

Now let's switch gears and head over to China. The varied systems of Chinese medicine are just as old—and just as complex—as the yoga systems from India. The basic underlying principle, however, is simple, and is depicted by the famous symbol of the yin/yang:

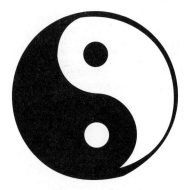

Chinese symbol depicting yin/yang forces.

The yin/yang represents a universal polarity. All things have a duality: night and day, dark and light, positive and negative, male and female, good and evil, sun and moon, hot and cold, soft and hard, etc.

But notice in the diagram that within each element (the black or the white) there's a small circle of the other element; each side contains the seed of the opposite. This is symbolic of the continuous process of change in the universe. Take yin to its extreme and it becomes yang, and vice versa. Learn to recognize that force of change in the world and the seed of the opposite in each moment and you will achieve balance. That's the underlying theme of t'ai chi healing.

The idea might be new to you. You're more likely to have heard of Traditional Chinese Medicine, or TCM. TCM refers to many Chinese systems, including acupuncture, acupressure, herbology, moxibustion, cupping, *t'ai chi ch'uan* (the exercise), and more. However, the term TCM isn't really used when discussing some of the more ancient systems, or some of which are still practiced today.

> **Finding Meaning**
>
> The Chinese martial art and exercise system, **t'ai chi ch'uan,** literally meaning "supreme ultimate fist," is based on the yin/yang principle of change. As a martial art, it uses softness to defeat an attacker by yielding to the incoming force and redirecting it, causing the attacker to defeat himself. Apart from its martial applications, it is a powerful and effective method of healthful exercise.

The ancient and modern systems aren't exactly the same but are both based on the principles of yin and yang. They all work to produce a balance within the yin and yang polarity of the energy matrix to promote health, longevity, and higher levels of awareness. In order to encompass all forms of Chinese healing—ancient and modern—I'm using the "umbrella" term t'ai chi healing.

We're using the term t'ai chi healing to refer to any system whose foundation is built on the t'ai chi, the supreme ultimate principle of yin and yang. This would refer to both ancient and modern Chinese medicine, traditional Japanese systems of shiatsu, macrobiotics, facial diagnosis, and all the other Asian physiognomy systems.

Now let's look at what some people call the scholars' yin/yang model: the t'ai chi t'u. It's a more detailed view of how the universe unfolded once the yin/yang polarity came into being. The words t'ai chi mean supreme ultimate (t'u means diagram).

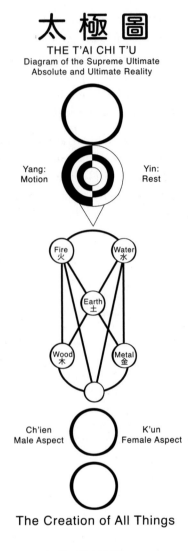

The T'ai Chi T'u.

Looking at the diagram, you'll see a sort of ladder between heaven and earth, which functions very similarly to the chakras, slowing down the faster energy from the higher levels to a frequency that the lower levels can handle. But while the chakras exist as a ladder within our own individual energy matrix, the t'ai chi t'u depicts a similar step-down transformer system within a more global energy bubble. Think of the t'ai chi t'u as a ladder within the WEB itself. The lowest level is our physical world, which the Chinese called the creation of all things; the higher levels are almost like different dimensions of energy. As you condition your own individual energy matrix—or upgrade it, as we've said—you can climb to higher and higher levels of the ladder. The highest level is what they called absolute reality and contains everything we can imagine, plus a lot of things we can't.

It's worth noting that in the diagram there are seven horizontal levels. The functions of these levels parallel the functions of the seven chakras *and* the systems in the body they relate to. Moreover, the overall goal of climbing the ladder to higher levels of emotional and spiritual awareness is the same within both paradigms.

No doubt you've heard of qi, the word used for energy in t'ai chi healing. Like prana in yoga, it goes by many different names, referring to different frequencies and functions.

Chinese characters are really pictures that tell a story. You just have to know how to read the different components that make up the picture. The word chi, for example, meaning life force or energy, is from the character in Chinese that means the steam that rises from a bowl of rice. The words t'ai chi means the ultimate central support, or destination, of the universe. The word chi is the same sound in English but not the same character or meaning in Chinese at all.

Qi moves through the energy matrix via a series of channels called meridians. The diagram on the next page shows the incredibly complex system of acupuncture meridians.

Traditionally there are 12 bi-lateral meridians (meaning that each meridian is found on either side of the body). Ten of them are named after a particular organ, such as the lungs, large intestine, stomach, spleen, and so on. Two of them, with rather unusual names (*triple warmer* and *pericardium*) refer to the broader functions of a whole system: the triple warmer refers to the endocrine glands or, more generally, the whole metabolic system, and the pericardium refers to the circulation of energy in the body, especially sexual energy. There are two additional meridians that circle the centerline of the body that help govern and control the energy flow in the other 12. They parallel the central line of the sushumna and chakras in yoga.

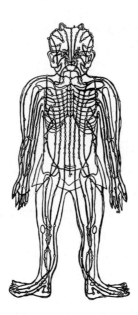

Master H'su Ch'ang's acupuncture meridians.

Keep in mind that when a meridian is labeled kidney or liver, it refers to the *energy* organ, not necessarily the physical one. While each of the meridians may have an effect on the physical organ, they can also connect with other, larger systems in the body: the gall bladder meridian to muscles, the liver meridian to the nervous system, and other meridians to blood or skin. That may help to explain how t'ai chi healing can treat many ailments that don't have anything to do with those 12 organs.

Another important thing to remember is that t'ai chi healing teaches us that there is really only one meridian, as the energy flows fluidly from one to the other throughout the body in one long loop; the division of names is almost for convenience.

Meridians form the connections between acupuncture points. There's an incredibly complex system of relationships known as the *five-element theory* that explains how energy flows between the meridians and their points in a variety of ways, which enable the expert t'ai chi healer to diagnose and treat complex ailments.

Finding Meaning

The five-element theory deals with relationships. The elements—fire, water, wood, earth, and metal—shouldn't be viewed as the physical things they represent. Think of them as different frequencies of energy found in nature. Together they form a model that's used in many areas of Chinese life, including medicine, martial arts, and music.

Kabbalah Healing

Kabbalah is the study of the ancient Jewish mystical tradition, and like yoga and t'ai chi healing, it's an incredibly vast and complex system. Let's get a handle on some of the basics so we can understand the significance to energy healing.

Imagine a time, before time even existed, when there was only an Infinite Oneness. Nothing else could exist and not be part of that Oneness. For purposes of seeing this clearly, imagine this Infinite Oneness as the box in the figure below. (I realize the irony of putting something infinite *inside of a box*, but trust me: it will help!)

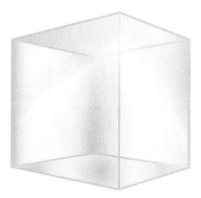

Ayn-Sof, The Infinite.

Then, one day (before there *were* days, remember!) this intelligent Oneness decided to create a bubble inside itself and allow for something else to exist there, inside the bubble.

What was inside the bubble? To put it simply—too simply, in fact—everything. The entire universe, both what we can see and what we can't see: galaxies, planets, gamma rays, X-rays, life forms, and even spirits and angels.

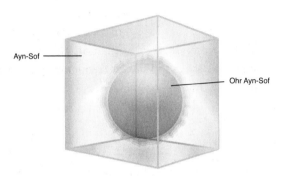

A Kabbalistic worldview.

And what's outside the bubble? Call it what you will: God, the Infinite Oneness, Brahm, or something else entirely. Kabbalah calls anything outside the bubble *Ayn-Sof*, the Infinite. Because what's outside the bubble is unknowable, let's focus our attention on what's knowable, the *inside* of the bubble.

Let's begin with light. Even though the bubble, by its very definition, is something separate from Ayn-Sof, it still exists within the Ayn-Sof, the Infinite. The light from the Ayn-Sof, which permeates the bubble, is called *Ohr Ayn-Sof,* the light of the Ayn-Sof (ohr is the Hebrew word for light). The Ohr Ayn-Sof is something we can encounter within our lives.

Finding Meaning

Ayn-Sof, the phrase Kabbalists use for God, literally means no end, or infinite. Ayn-Sof is unknowable unity. **Ohr Ayn-Sof** is the slower light that fills the inside of the bubble of our universe, the WEB. Remember this: Ayn-Sof is everything, the Infinite Oneness. Ohr Ayn-Sof is the slower, differentiated light that exists only inside the bubble.

Remember when we discussed chakras, we said that some kind of step-down transformer system is necessary to bring the faster light down to our slower-frequency reality. The same thing is true of the light from the Ayn-Sof. That light needs to be slowed down before we can access it.

In Kabbalistic teaching, there are four major worlds, or dimensions, called *olamot*. When most people think of dimensions, they think in terms of space and time. However, in physics, a dimension is also defined by velocity, and because we've been talking about faster and slower energies, dimension is the perfect word to explain the olamot. They're worlds within worlds, each operating on a slower and slower frequency, the lowest (or innermost) being our physical world.

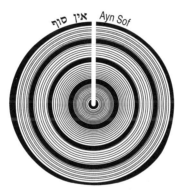

Olamot are major worlds or dimensions.

It's helpful to think of the other three worlds—the ones within the bubble that operate on higher frequencies than our physical world—as what we've been calling the WEB. Through meditation, upgrading of our energy matrix (or chakras), etc., we're able to access the higher frequency energies of the Ohr Ayn-Sof.

That brings us to another essential yet amazingly complicated concept: the energy building blocks of the universe. There are 10 different energies called *sefirot* that comprise 10 distinct aspects of knowledge that are the foundation of creation. Don't think of them like electricity running through a wire; they're more like intelligences.

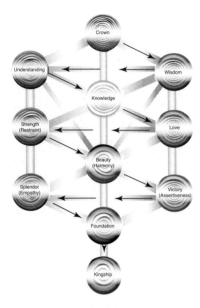

The Kabbalistic Tree of Life—sefirot.

All four olamot are built from the building blocks of the sefirot, and the energy of the sefirot is found in each of the worlds. The combination of the sefirot and the olamot create an elaborate array of step-down transformers of the infinite light in the WEB.

Olamot means worlds in Hebrew. The world is something you can see. But there's an interesting aspect to the singular form of the word; olam can also mean invisible, what you *cannot* see. It's the perfect word to describe our universe, our WEB, because it includes everything you see *and* everything you don't see.

Sefirot are the 10 forces that have built the universe. Metaphorically, they are the 10 fingers of the Infinite Creator, and they exist in each of us. Sefirah is related to other English and Hebrew words: cipher, the primary 10 numbers; sapphire, a luminous jewel; sippur, a story; and say'fer, book. The sefirot are the 10 intelligent, radiant stories of the world's book of life.

The sefirot exist in each of the olamot in the same way that scales in music can exist on many octaves. Think of a piano and visualize the different octaves of music. Each octave has do, re, mi; it's just that each higher-note do is a super-harmonic of the other dos beneath it. That is, it's the same vibratory note, only one octave higher because it has a higher frequency.

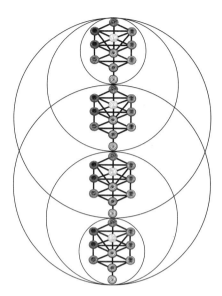

Each of the olamot with their sefirot.

In addition to the sefirot being in each of the universal, macrocosmic olamot, they also exist as a microcosmic ladder inside each of us. We are each at the base of a ladder that enables us to climb as high as our potential, aspirations, and efforts can take us.

One last point: in addition to the 10 sefirot themselves, there are also sefirotic strings that connect the sefirot together. Those 22 strings, which correspond to the 22 letters of the Hebrew alphabet, are the conduits through which the slowed-down energy flows from the higher sefirot so it can be received by the lower receivers on the ladder.

Our goal is to prepare the microcosmic ladder within each of us (the energy matrix) and use it to climb through the higher and higher levels of the WEB. Think of your energy matrix as a chariot you must prepare for the journey that is your life. Preparation is the key: if the body, energy, mind, character, feelings, and thoughts aren't properly prepared through study and practice (which from a Kabbalistic point of view, is accomplished by living one's life according to the precepts within the Torah, the Jewish bible), we can short-circuit the process. Remember, it took only one small O-ring to bring the Space Shuttle to disaster.

In science, the idea that the same model can manifest over and over at lesser degrees is what is called a *fractal*, a shape that can be split into parts, each of which is a reduced-size copy of the whole. We see this in nature in clouds, snowflakes, lightning, blood vessels, and trees. We also see it in the repeated presence of the sefirot inside the WEB. As above, so below.

What These Systems Have in Common

We now have a very basic and simplified understanding of three diverse approaches to understanding and encountering life. Clearly, each of these bodies of ancient knowledge requires reading volumes and volumes to fully comprehend it. And even then, there will be confusion and questions left unanswered. We're looking at the big picture to develop a richer perspective and understanding of energy healing as a whole. Let's summarize what we've learned so far, using our new vocabulary:

Our knowable world, both physical and spiritual, exists within a WEB, a worldwide energy bubble, filled with Prana, Chi, Ohr Ayn-Sof, the light of the Infinite.

Each of our bodies exists within an energy matrix, a field of energy that has its own anatomy and energy distribution system (nadis, meridians, internal sefirotic strings), just as the physical body does.

The energy matrix is a chariot that enables us, once upgraded and prepared, to rise to higher and higher levels and bring wisdom and healing energy back down to this world.

And where does this energy come from? From the WEB, the worldwide energy bubble, an ocean of energy all around us, a supreme ultimate hierarchy.

Like the microcosm of our personal energy matrix, the WEB is a ladder, bringing the highest energy and wisdom down to us through a series of step-down transformers (dimensions, olamot, worlds, chakras).

Our energy matrix receives the energy and channels it through to wherever it is needed. The WEB is a macrocosmic version of the microcosm of the energy matrix.

Pretty amazing, right? Here we are, describing three incredibly diverse cultures, but when viewed from the top of the mountain, they share very similar paradigms. In each culture, the seers, mystics, and prophets looked more deeply into reality than the rest of us normally do. They described them differently, and came up with different explanations, but no matter where they lived, an atom was still an atom.

No matter what your culture, your anatomy and physiology work the same. And no matter how your culture describes it, your personal energy matrix and the ocean of energy within which we all reside remain the same.

If you're a student or practitioner of one of the myriad of energy healing systems we haven't mentioned, go back and take a second look at your system. Whether you're a student of Polynesian Huna, a Native American shaman, or a cranio-sacral therapist, look at your system's paradigm, the energy world within which you function, and see if the energy matrix and WEB model offer some clarity, once you get past the words. Perhaps it will be a small step in bringing us all together to be part of the healing that's needed in the world.

Essential Takeaways

- There are many similarities between the different energy systems when we learn to use our common vocabulary and look past the words.

- Yoga healing describes a picture of chakras, prana, nadis, and kundalini.

- T'ai chi healing describes a world of qi and meridians, and five-element theory.

- Kabbalah outlines a world of olamot, sefirot, Ohr Ayn-Sof, and a worldwide energy bubble of conscious light.

- Kabbalah describes a world with a ladder enabling us to climb to higher levels of consciousness, and a chariot to help us to do so (the energy matrix).

chapter 3

Scientific Perspectives in Energy Healing

Studying the science of energy healing

Measuring the effects of thoughts, words, and feelings

Altered brain waves in energy healing

A scientific theory of how energy healing works

Energy healing and the Age of Aquarius

After looking at some of the ancient systems, you have to wonder: this is all fine and good, but does any of this stuff stand up to scientific scrutiny?

We may not have a single scientific theory that explains it all, but then, physicists continue to debate theories of how the quantum sub-atomic universe works, also. Energy healing, by its nature, is happening somewhere in the quantum universe, too, so a full understanding will surface in time. But as we begin to explore some of the science behind energy healing, I think you'll find that there's more evidence out there than you thought.

Science Begins to Engage Energy Healing

There are a few groundbreaking scientists who can help us begin to understand how energy healing might work. Taken together, they provide a working theory that will enable us to continue our exploration of energy, and to further combine the ideas behind ancient and modern systems. Let's look at just a sample of some of these groundbreakers.

Harold Saxton Burr

For over 30 years, Dr. Harold Saxton Burr, Professor Emeritus of Anatomy at Yale's School of Medicine, and his associates were able to measure electromagnetic fields of life—he called them L-fields—around living forms: humans, animals, trees, plants, and even lower life forms. He believed those L-fields were the organizing mechanism that built, maintained, and repaired the physical forms of all living things.

This work was done in the early part of the twentieth century, and no doubt there are labs that are now attempting to corroborate his work with better technology. But with relatively simple, specially designed voltmeters, he was able to detect and measure electrical changes indicative of many health benchmarks and problems. He was able to detect, for example, internal physiological changes such as the beginning of women's menstrual cycles. He saw energy shifts while wounds were healing and was even able to predict which might grow into stronger and healthier plants by measuring the electrical output of seeds.

In *Design for Destiny*, a book partly documenting Dr. Burr's work, Edward Russell wrote that " … the L-field is the controlling, organizing force of the living form—an electrical matrix which molds living matter. It is also another illustration of the important fact that the field *anticipates* physical conditions." Energy healers have been able to replicate that sensing of health problems for millennia, and without a special voltmeter.

Preventative Healing

It's not unusual for an energy healer to read the energy matrix of the patient and be able to sense a problem even before any physical signs manifest. It's an aspect of the "as above, so below" principle. If the healer can eliminate the energy block above, the imbalance may be prevented from ever becoming a physical symptom below.

Years ago, I did some energy work on a close friend of my brother's. She had been suffering with a persistent cough and chest soreness—probably from the coughing—that had been unresponsive to medication for months. I worked with her for three sessions to break up the energy blocks that hadn't allowed her body to heal itself. I also taught her some basic energy massage that she could do on herself to help the process along. The cough, unchanged for half a year, cleared up in just three days.

During a session, I asked her about something I felt as I scanned her energy matrix. There seemed to be an energy anomaly in her intestines. She said she'd never had a problem there, so I dismissed it and didn't work on it any further. Soon after, she began having a variety of intestinal problems; her doctor said they were probably related to whatever had caused her mother's colitis, which I didn't know about. Weeks of medications and suppositories got rid of the problem.

As with Burr's predictive L-fields, the energy matrix had manifested the problem before the body did. Too bad we hadn't discovered it sooner and broken up the energy blocks in the matrix, possibly preventing the unpleasantness of the treatment.

Dr. Emoto's Water Crystals

Another pioneer, Masaru Emoto of Japan was able to develop a method for photographing water crystals in a way that has never been done before, using a powerful dark-field microscope attached to a high-speed camera. He discovered that our thoughts, words, and emotions were able to affect water molecules enough to change the shape of the frozen crystals. Looking at the shape and aesthetic of the water crystals he photographed, he was able to see that clear spring water made more beautiful crystals than polluted water. Well, no surprise there!

Then he took a bottle of water, wrapped it with a piece of paper with a positive thought on it—love, gratitude, or something similar—and saw that the crystals from that water had bright, beautiful, and complex patterns. When he took another bottle of the same type of water and tied a negative thought around it—you make me sick; I will kill you—the crystals were "incomplete, asymmetrical and dull."

Notice the words or thoughts beneath the water in each of the following photos. The ones taken before and after a Buddhist healing prayer are of great significance in our study of energy healing; these photos are almost enough to convince anyone of the power and effect of thought in energy healing.

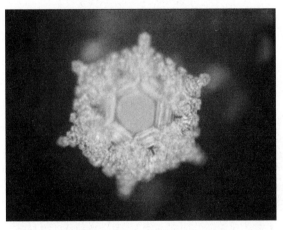

Love and gratitude (reprinted with permission of Office Masaru Emoto, LLC.).

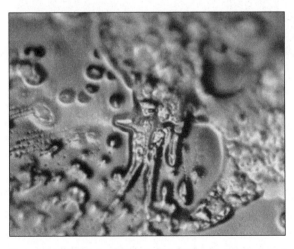

You make me sick; I will kill you (reprinted with permission of Office Masaru Emoto, LLC.).

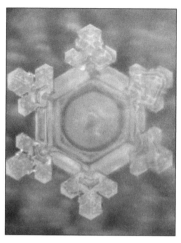

Thank you (reprinted with permission of
Office Masaru Emoto, LLC.).

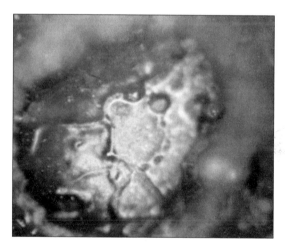

Lake water before prayer (reprinted with permission of
Office Masaru Emoto, LLC.).

We'll be discussing using water in energy healing later on. In the meantime, think about this: our bodies are 70–90 percent water. If negative thoughts have a proven impact on water, imagine what's happening to your body when someone sends negative thoughts your way! Or more importantly, think about what's happening when we have negative thoughts about ourselves!

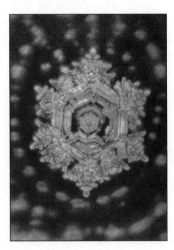

Lake water after Buddhist healing prayer (reprinted with permission of Office Masaru Emoto, LLC.).

Messages from Water

MISC.

In 2005, Dr. Emoto's Peace Project was announced at The Spiritual Dimensions of Science and Consciousness Subcommittee at the United Nations. It aims to educate children about how thoughts, words, and feelings can affect water and also themselves. The goal of the project is to distribute 650 million free copies of their children's book, *Messages from Water,* to children age 3 through 12, throughout the world over the next 10 years.

The Holographic Universe

Now let's look at a theory from the world of quantum physics that comes very close to describing what we call the WEB, the ocean of energy that surrounds us and is the essence of our unseen reality.

A relatively new idea that's gaining acceptability in quantum physics is that the entire universe is a *hologram.*

Finding Meaning

A **hologram** is a 3-D image produced by wave interference patterns and stored on a 2-D surface. Unlike a photographic negative, where you can see the actual image in reverse, the 2-D surface of the hologram looks like random wave patterns. But when a laser illuminates the surface, a 3-D image is projected from it.

The little holograms on your credit cards have the appearance of shiny three-dimensional (3-D) objects. But really, all the information in that little hologram is on a two-dimensional (2-D) piece of plastic and merely seems to be projecting a 3-D image.

Scientists today are hypothesizing that all the information in our universe is projected from the 2-D inner surface of a giant dome (a WEB?) and our reality, our entire universe, is a holographic projection within that dome. For *Star Trek* fans, this resembles the holodeck on the Starship *Enterprise*. The room was an empty space and the computer created a 3-D solid reality within its 2-D walls.

Think back to the Kabbalistic model discussed in the previous chapter: the Ayn-Sof, the Infinite One, created a bubble inside Himself and utilized sefirotic energies to project all the dimensions of our reality within that bubble. If you can get past the difference in language, it seems that in this case, science and mysticism are saying something quite similar.

This is just one theory, but it does get you thinking. Both scientists and mystics are on a continual search to explain a reality that's more than what it appears to be, and we're likely to see more overlap like this in the future.

Brain Waves

Here is an example of energy healing science at its most basic! My first venture into a laboratory for anything related to energy healing happened in my early 20s, almost by accident.

In Chapter 1, I discussed brain waves and altered states of consciousness. In those days I wasn't paying much attention to them; I was busy with martial arts and yoga training, mastering certain skills of movement, breathing, and focus. The fact that they might be altering my brain waves wasn't something I thought about.

One of my beginner martial arts students, Jack, was studying psychology at Clemson University. He asked me if I would be part of an experiment he was doing. I didn't understand it completely at the time, but I agreed.

Jack put me in a room as small as a closet, wired me up to a machine that measured brain waves, and asked me to relax while he took some readings.

Then he asked my young wife, Lillian, to enter the room for a minute and do whatever she could to get me into an excited, waking beta state. After she left, he wanted to see how long it would take for me to re-relax and regain whatever brain wave patterns I'd had before she came in.

The experiment went along just fine. It was quite easy to see the changes in the squiggly lines on the readout, though I had no idea what I was looking at. But as Jack looked at the readouts, he got a worried look on his face. He was seeing a type of brain wave he'd never studied about or seen. He was worried that I had something wrong with me health-wise, and that he might have discovered it by accident. He took the readings directly to his professor.

Jack arrived at the next karate class smiling and bewildered. Apparently, I had generated a more perfect alpha wave than either he or his professor had ever seen. Apparently, intense training in martial arts and yoga had given me more control over my brain waves than I had expected. The alpha range of brain wave frequency of 8 hz is the most conducive to effective energy healing, something I didn't understand till years later when I met Dr. Andrija Puharich.

Dr. Puharich's Theory of Healing

The years I spent with the late Dr. Andrija Puharich, MD, opened my eyes and expanded my paradigm in a variety of ways. This gentle-hearted neurologist/researcher/author spent many decades studying bona-fide healers and psychics all over the planet. He sought a unified scientific theory to explain the many phenomena he'd observed and made some significant progress.

As a physician, energy healing was his first love. His work and thinking inspired me to move forward in my own efforts to understand and practice energy healing.

Here are some of the ideas and pioneers to whom he introduced me.

Tesla's Model of the World

The first time I entered Dr. Puharich's office I couldn't help but notice a fantastic electrical model on his desk. It was a light bulb of sorts, about

8 inches across. It had what looked like a filament in the middle: a small black sphere, about an inch or so in diameter. Between the black sphere and the outside of the bulb were a few dozen sparks that looked like lightning.

Puharich said it was a model of the earth developed by Nikola Tesla, one of the great minds of the early twentieth century. Puharich was a major authority on Tesla, his interest sparked (no pun intended) by the fact that they were both of Serbo-Croatian descent.

Nikola Tesla

Tesla invented alternating current, a discovery that changed the world. With AC current, you didn't need giant generators on every corner, as Thomas Edison's DC current demanded. He also invented countless other devices, including the Tesla coil. The list of his inventions and patents—not to mention his extreme obsessive-compulsive behavior—has been a subject of interest for biographers and filmmakers.

"How is this a model for the earth?" I asked. He explained that the black ball at the center represented the earth, which is negatively charged. The outside bubble was the ionosphere, which is positively charged. Between the earth's core and the ionosphere is a 2-billion-volt electrical potential. The lightning bolts were the natural discharge in the giant battery in which we lived. He told me that at any one second, there were at least 500 real lightning bolts discharging all over the earth.

And that's what healers do, according to Puharich. They tap into the energy around them and channel it into the healing of others. He asked me to put my finger on the top of the glass bubble. I did, and something amazing happened. All the lightning bolts seemed to converge into one between my finger and the center of the globe. I could feel the buzz in my fingertip.

Puharich said that just as my finger was able to focus the energy inside the globe, healers focus the energy within themselves. They tap into the energy around them, draw it into their own energy matrix, and aim it at the patient for healing.

All of the energies that Puharich was talking about were in the extremely low-frequency range, about 1–100 hz. He called them E.L.F. for short.

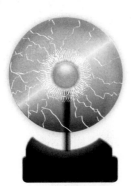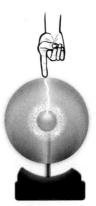

Tesla Globe alone and with fingertip

The Telsa globe reacts when touched.

Be careful if you buy one of those little Tesla-ball models. I've found you can spend way too much time having fun with them and not enough time learning the lessons of energy healing. It's important to have fun, but remember: moderation, students, moderation!

E.L.F. and Energy Healing Theory

The following information is from the cheat sheet on E.L.F. Puharich prepared for me and other nonscientists.

- In spite of their ultra weak power, E.L.F. fields, also known as scalar fields, can affect biological systems in a most profound way.

- E.L.F. fields can go through anything and are nonattenuating, meaning they don't get weaker with distance. Only DNA, particularly in the brain, stops E.L.F. fields.

- The beneficial frequencies of E.L.F. are in the range of 7–9 hz (or cycles per second). This frequency is related to the 8 hz magnetic fields from the sun and the 8 hz frequency of the earth.

- This 8 hz frequency is also related to the Schumann resonance, a term commonly found in energy healing systems referring to the 7.82 hz "heartbeat" of the earth.

Our DNA, the genetic code in our cells that defines our traits and is the source of any mutations that may lead to disease, is like a spiral staircase. The steps joining the two sides of the stairway (helices) are complicated molecules called bases which pair together to form the steps. At the center of those steps, you'll always find hydrogen atoms interacting between two "base pairs" to bind them together.

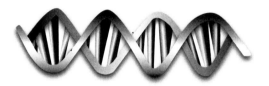

The DNA double helix.

Imagine DNA as a musical keyboard. If you were to stretch out a strand to its full 1–2 meter length, each gene would be like a different note or key. Pushing keys allows you to activate or deactivate functions or effects in the body by triggering or eliminating specific gene activity. In this way, the right combination of key-strokes can slow or eliminate disease as well as enhance the body's natural ability to heal itself.

In the presence of certain protein substances in the nuclei of the cell, E.L.F. fields interact with the DNA molecule itself. Because each gene is frequency-specific, meaning that individual frequencies can change the programming of the cell, the E.L.F. fields can actually turn on or off any gene.

For example, in lab tests, one frequency was shown to cause cancer in rats in two days, but another reversed the process. One frequency can cause depression in humans by causing the release of chemicals (cholinergic neuropeptides) in the brain, while still another can cause anxiety. These things can be done from as far away as the other side of the planet with the correct equipment.

stay Grounded

Warning—serious science ahead! If you're more interested in the energy part of this, and the science just makes your head spin, that's okay. You don't necessarily need to understand how external magnetic fields can control biological spin-spin proton-proton coupling constants in DNA, RNA, RNA transferases, and hydrons (H_2O). Don't worry; I don't understand all of it, either. The important thing to know is that E.L.F. fields can produce powerful effects on biological systems.

According to the U.S. Navy, which conducted testing for seven years, the following effects of E.L.F. have been reproduced in numerous laboratory tests:

Alter the behavior of cells, tissues, organs, and organisms

Alter hormone levels

Alter the reaction time of irreversible chemical processes

Alter cell chemistry

Alter time perception in animals and humans

Induce sleep in animals

Inhibit/enhance bone growth

Inhibit/enhance cell de-differentiation

Inhibit/enhance protein kinase production

Inhibit/enhance mRNA (messenger RNA) synthesis and process

Affect the immune process

Affect calcium ion bonding in cells

Suppress cAMP (cyclic-AMP) production

Destroy or rupture cells

Entrain human brain waves

Entrain the DNA transcription process

Cause defects and alterations in embryos

Cause up to six times higher fetus mortality rate in lab animals than in controls

Cause sterility in male animals

Slow the aging process of cells

Cause noninvasive genetic engineering

Cure certain diseases by altering their E.L.F. frequency

Here's the thing: E.L.F. fields can affect human organisms big-time. If we could learn to generate E.L.F. brain wave signals ourselves with the intention to heal, imagine what we could accomplish.

Putting the E.L.F. Theory into Healing Practice

How do you focus your mind to prepare to send out frequency-specific E.L.F. healing energy and, once in that state, how do you connect to someone else's frequency for a healing encounter?

To put it in the terms of our common vocabulary, we need our energy matrix to log on to the WEB. To do that we want to get our energy matrix in tune with the heartbeat of the earth; we want a relaxed, deep alpha brain wave, around 8 hz, so we're at the same frequency as the 2-billion-volt electrical potential of the planet. But the mind is busy with life; the two hemispheres of the brain are like boxers in a ring, continuing to battle to decide who's in charge: the cognitive, logical side or the creative, intuitive side.

In repeated lab experiments, Puharich observed that with a simple method called ocular divergence (turn to Chapter 14 for further information), you can learn to uncouple the hemispheres of the brain to send those boxers back to their corners for a time-out. Now that your mind is quiet you can reach the alpha state and, once there, focus on the energy matrix and ground yourself, or root (explained in Chapter 14), into the earth's energy field.

Now that we've reached alpha, we can consider how to connect to someone else's frequency for healing.

Think of a cell phone. If I want to talk to someone on the other side of the world, I take my cell phone and call his number—his frequency-specific address. My voice is converted to energy signals that bounce off a tower, go to a satellite in space, transfer to another satellite on the other side of the planet, drop back down to a receiving dish in his country, and go to my friend's cell phone, where it's converted back into the sound of my voice. He answers his phone, I speak, and he recognizes my voice. Unbelievable—it almost sounds more "out there" than remote energy healing does.

In the case of healing, how does one human entrain the frequency of the other so that healing energy can be transmitted? To use our cell phone analogy, how does the healer get the phone number for the patient's energy matrix?

Puharich wired up both the healer and the patient to EEGs, brain wave measurement devices much more sophisticated than the one Jack used in Clemson. He discovered, and demonstrated repeatedly, that once the healer was in a healing state of mind (8 hz), and came physically close to the patient, the patient's brain wave was entrained by the healer's. Entrainment means that the brain waves of the healer and the patient begin to vibrate at the same frequency, in this case, that of the healer. The healer was able to *phase-lock* with the patient on that frequency and send healing energy.

Finding Meaning

Phase-locking with a patient is very similar to the way a tuning fork vibrates a piano string when they're at the same frequency. One frequency capturing or entraining another and locking into it—one wave phase-locking the other—is referred to as rhythmic entrainment. In energy healing, you can do the same thing with the focused intention of your mind.

I saw it in the lab and have been wired up and tested myself. Watching the digital and print read-out as it was happening, and seeing the two brain waves synchronize, was mind-blowing.

Now that we've achieved that relaxed 8 hz alpha state and have phase-locked with the patient, we can transmit specific frequencies of E.L.F. scalar fields to the DNA in the patient's body. The diseased cells get the new information and programming. In a perfect world, that's your goal. And, more often than you might think, it happens just like that.

String Theory

Back in the 1980s, Steven M. Phillips wrote a book called *Extra-Sensory Perception of Quarks*. In it he reported that over a century before, a number of theosophists—a religious philosophical group that focused on mystical studies and occult experiences—got together and psychically viewed what they thought was an atom and drew pictures of what they saw. Phillips compared those old drawings with some current visual ideas of quantum physics' *string theory*, an idea of how things really look and work in the sub-atomic world. He discovered that the pictures were very similar.

Finding Meaning

String theory, which proposes that the universe is comprised of and filled with subtle and tiny energy strings, may be the missing link between general relativity—the science of the galactic universe—and quantum mechanics, the science of the very small sub-atomic universe. Einstein spent the last 30 years of his life looking for such a unified theory.

According to Puharich, the basic hydrogen atom is the most omnipresent element in the universe and is at the center of each of the steps in the DNA double helix staircase. Those atoms, he believed, are what actually receive the E.L.F. messages from the healer and push the keys in the DNA keyboard to make energy healing happen. Essentially, the hydrogen atoms are receiver-transmitters that can communicate with each other.

He drew a picture of a hydrogen atom, with a very large proton and a small electron orbiting it. Then he added some circles inside the proton. Inside each proton he sketched three quarks, very small sub-atomic particles.

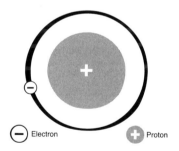

Depiction of a hydrogen atom.

The three quarks were attached by strings. Inside each of them he drew three more little circles and joined them by little strings as well, which he called monopoles because they're so small that, unlike magnets, they have only one pole. The nine little circles (three bound quarks) inside the proton, plus the one unbound electron spinning around it, constitute the 10-dimensional essence that impacts virtually everything and is the basis for all energy healing.

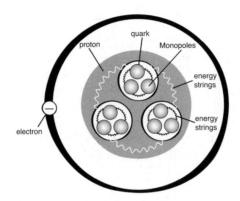

Hydrogen atom with quarks, monopoles, and strings.

Science and Ancient Healing

Strange as it may seem, there's a reason why quarks and hydrogen atoms are entering into our discussion of energy healing.

If we take that round bag model of the proton (the quarks and the strings) and straighten it out, it looks a lot like the diagram of the t'ai chi t'u and the sefirotic tree of life in Chapter 2. And it has the same 10 components and 7 horizontal levels we saw in the chakras.

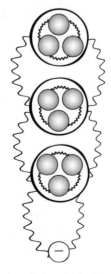

A vertical rendering of a hydrogen atom.

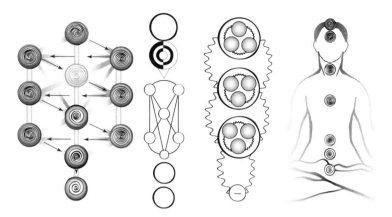

Comparative paradigms.

What I'm suggesting is this: throughout history, seers, psychics, and mystics, in altered states, have peeked into the mysteries of life and seen the same picture but used different words, images, and models to describe it. Now we're seeing that theoretical physicists are joining the mix, adding their completed model of how life works. It's the oldest story there is—and also the newest.

I've always found that the combination of Puharich's quantum physics and the energy matrix/WEB paradigm provided a workable hypothesis to predict what might happen during a healing. As time goes on, I believe physicists and mystics will continue to come closer together with a more complete explanation. In the meantime, we can do the work of energy healing even if we aren't 100 percent certain how it works.

The Aquarian Paradigm Shift in Energy Healing

The idea of the "dawning of the Age of Aquarius," made popular by the song from the musical *Hair*, refers to an ancient idea that approximately every 2,100 years, the world shifts from the influence of one particular constellation's impact on life on Earth and moves on to another. That influence affects healing, communication, education, and virtually every human endeavor.

There are two major cycles in astrology, personal and cosmic. Most people are familiar with the normal personal astrological cycle (in which Aquarius is the month before Pisces). There is also a cosmic 25,000 cycle: Every 2,100 years, a new root-race begins, bringing the planet under the influence of a different constellation. In the cosmic cycle, the signs are reversed, which is why the Age of Pisces came before the Age of Aquarius.

The symbol of the Age of Pisces (the last two millennia) was the fish, a water sign. If you look at the way medicine has been conducted for the last two millennia (pre-modern medicine), a lot was based on water: water cures, soaks in hot springs and salts, potions, elixirs, etc.

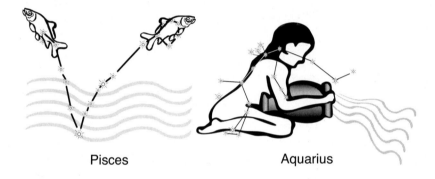

Pisces   Aquarius

Representations of Pisces and Aquarius.

The symbol of Aquarius is a water-bearer. Interestingly, all the images of the Aquarian constellation show waves of water being poured out of an urn. So Aquarius is to be an age of waves.

In the last 150 years—the dawn of modern medicine—X-rays, ultra-sound, MRIs, CAT-scans, lasers, radiation, and computerized procedures that require electrical waves, not water—have all been introduced. And this is just beginning as we make a gradual entry into the Aquarian Age. Who knows what energy wonders will be part of conventional medicine by the end of the twenty-first century?

Perhaps the Age of Aquarius will usher in a time when conventional medicine and energy healing will draw closer together. They both share the same goal—to heal—and if they can continue to grow and learn from each other, the possibilities are limitless.

Essential Takeaways

- There's a burgeoning science behind how we can train our energy matrix to phase-lock with the beat of the earth, tapping into its vast energy reservoir.

- Our thoughts, words, and feelings affect both the energy matrix and the physical world, as seen by their effect on water crystals and L-fields.

- We can now measure the connection between a healer and a patient, creating a vibratory line of communication between them.

- A healer can impact the energy matrix of a patient by directing E.L.F. scalar fields at it, which are captured by the hydrogen atoms in DNA.

- E.L.F. fields can cause a myriad of biological changes by pushing the specific keys on the DNA keyboard.

- Energy healing and conventional medicine will, through scientific understanding and a desire for personal and world healing, come closer together.

- Side by side, the diagrams of some of the ancient systems look remarkably similar to those of quantum physics.

chapter 4

Stress and Energy Healing

How stress affects our minds and bodies

The fight-or-flight response in the twenty-first century

The energy matrix and the stress-block cycle

Stress causes problems. That seems like an obvious statement; it's something we all know. But it's also the most overt example of how energy can affect our physical bodies. By understanding the energy component in the body's stress cycle, we can begin to see that this is the perfect place to begin our exploration of how, why, and when energy healing works.

Stress and Disease

Stress is clearly the single-greatest threat to our lives today. In the accelerated world we live in, there's no greater cause of unhappiness, physical suffering, or even death than our mishandling of stress.

According to the American Heart Association, over 30 percent of the annual death rate in the United States is caused by stroke or heart disease, both of which have been linked to stress. Starting to see just how important stress management is to our daily lives, and how energy healing can help us?

Stress as Applied to Humans

The word *stress* began as an engineering term, meaning a force brought to bear on a system that tends to distort it. For example, too heavy a load on the roof of a building (i.e., too much stress) will cause the building to collapse. The word stressor is used to describe that force or event. Both terms have more recently been applied to the human condition.

Read through the list of diseases or symptoms. Every one of them is caused or, at the very least, aggravated by stress.

- Allergies
- Arteriosclerosis
- Arthritis
- Atopic dermatitis (Eczema)
- Backache
- Cancer
- Colitis
- Constipation
- Depression
- Diabetes
- Diarrhea
- Dizziness
- Epilepsy
- Headaches
- Heart problems
- Hypertension (high blood pressure)
- Hypoglycemia
- Insomnia
- Lessened immunity to infection
- Menstrual disorders
- Migraines
- Nervous breakdown
- Shoulder/neck pain
- Stroke
- Thyroid disorders
- Ulcers

Can energy healing help combat these often-debilitating diseases? Absolutely. The first step is to understand how stress works so we can take steps to minimize its harmful effects right from the start.

The Physiology of Stress

What happens to the body under stress? During a stressful event the two parts of the brain—the thinking part (the cortex) and the automatic part (the limbic system)—produce physiological changes. The cortex perceives an event as dangerous, or stressful. Then the limbic system responds to the danger by activating the body's defense system.

The autonomic nervous system is in charge of keeping your internal organs and systems running smoothly. It's also your first line of defense against any threats to your body, external or internal. It has two parts: the sympathetic branch, which evokes the fight-or-flight response to deal with stressful or threatening events in your life, and the parasympathetic branch, which evokes the relaxation response and keeps you calm when there are no immediate threats.

The fight-or-flight response prepared primitive humans to run from life-threatening danger or to mobilize their defenses to confront it. Do we stay and fight the saber-toothed tiger, or do we run away from it?

During the fight-or-flight response, when stressful stimuli bring about the arousal of the sympathetic branch of the autonomic nervous system, what happens to you?

- The hypothalamus activates the pituitary gland.

- The pituitary releases *ACTH* into the bloodstream.

Finding Meaning

ACTH, or Adrenocorticotropic hormone, is produced and secreted by the pituitary gland. A major component of the hypothalamic-pituitary-adrenal axis, it tells the adrenal glands to mobilize the body to deal with stress.

- ACTH activates the adrenal glands, which release catecholamines, hormones produced by stress, such as adrenaline, noradrenalin, and cortisol.

This, in turn, causes the following:

- The blood supply is diverted from the internal organs to the brain and skeletal muscles, providing energy for quick reacting and vigorous physical activity. Basically, it gives you that boost of energy you need to fight or run.

- The pupils dilate and the eardrums tighten, making you more sensitive to gradations of light and sound. This is a good thing if you're threatened by a real, imminent danger and you need to fight or run.

- The heart rate speeds up and the blood pressure becomes elevated (moving your blood more quickly through your circulatory system) to provide you with the oxygen you need to—you guessed it—fight or run.

- Your breathing becomes more rapid, providing increased availability of oxygen, enabling you to have the energy to fight or run.

- You perspire, maintaining optimum temperature for your muscles to fight or run.

Once the stressful event passes, the parasympathetic branch of the autonomic nervous system kicks in, bringing the body back to a balanced state by a process called the relaxation response. An opposite set of parasympathetic chemicals are released to bring the elevated responses back down and return you to equilibrium.

Stress and the Body-Mind

Before any of those physical things happen, though, one key component must occur: your mind has to tell your body that an event is stressful. Events themselves are completely neutral; it's how we perceive, understand, and react to them that make them stressful or not. A stack of unpaid bills never killed anyone, but the anxiety we allow ourselves to feel over those bills can be catastrophic.

And it's not the same for everyone. Your individual experiences have conditioned you to perceive stressors differently from the next person. You might even perceive a stressor where none exists because of your personal experiences.

For example, if a mugger suddenly attacks you on the street, you could respond in a number of ways. If you're a trained fighter, you might try to defend yourself. Or you could yell for help. Or run. Or you could freeze in your tracks: fight or flight or freeze in fright.

Fight-or-Flight Connections

Suppose that when you were a kid, your dad decided to teach you to swim by the drastic sink-or-swim method. He tossed you into a cold lake—and you sank under the water for what seemed like an eternity. Ever since then you've had an irrational fear of deep water. Whenever you're faced with a situation that calls for swimming, you unconsciously react with fight or flight based on your response to an incident that took place 10 or 20 years ago.

Whether your reaction is generated by the conscious mind (as with the mugger) or the subconscious (as with swimming), your body and mind are inseparably linked when it comes to the fight-or-flight response.

This shows that our psychological and emotional responses to stressors are just as important as our physical responses.

Moreover—and this is a key point—your body can't always tell the difference between real stress and imagined stress. Compare these two scenarios:

Scenario A: You're walking down the street and a mugger with a weapon jumps out at you. This evokes the fight-or-flight response. And that's a good thing.

Scenario B: You have a friend who likes playing tricks, and one night as you're approaching your home, he jumps out at you from behind a bush.

Two things immediately come to mind regarding Scenario B: first, you may want to reconsider your choice of friends. But second, and far more important, is that your body can't tell the difference between those two encounters, one potentially life-threatening and the other just a bad joke.

If our perceptions and paradigm determine whether an event is stressful, then with the proper motivation and training, we can control our emotional responses to stress. And if we can do that, we can learn to use stress to provide the positive stimuli for assertive and creative action. You may be wondering how stress can be a positive thing. If you've ever heard people say they work well under pressure, you already know the answer.

Where the System Breaks Down

The fight-or-flight system was designed for life-threatening situations like an enemy from the next village or a violent act of nature. These stressors usually happened infrequently, but when they did, they were real dangers.

The thing about immediate physical threats is that they pass. But nowadays, in our busy, civilized world, the things that stress us out don't just go away like a wild animal moving on. News reports, chemicals in your foods, electromagnetic signals of all types, bosses who thrive on your pain, traffic …. Each one of those stressors pumps chemicals into your body to raise your blood pressure and pulse rate to prepare you to fight or run as if a real threat to your survival was happening. If you were able to physically fight or run, thereby eliminating these stressors, it would provide closure and resolution. This in turn would stop the production of stress hormones that are being secreted by your body. Such definitive action (eliminating the stressor) would also evoke your relaxation response, and bring you back to a state of equilibrium.

The trouble is, you can't physically fight or run most of the time. And the fact that we're so much more sedentary than our ancestors doesn't help. If your boss barks at you, you certainly can't fight him, and going for a quick jog around the block would not get him out of your life (or even get him to be nicer). When we can't fight or run, we're left with ongoing stressors (sometimes sub-consciously) that keep pouring stress hormones into our bodies. And with all those hormones constantly in circulation within our bodies, responding to ongoing real or imagined threats every day, the body is unable to return to a balanced state.

Deeper Connections

Modern stressors are much more subtle than the old-time ones, but they still trigger the fight-or-flight response. The boss yelling at you isn't immediately life-threatening, but if he's angry at you, you could get fired. Then you'll run out of money and then you'll starve … and starvation is a real stressor! That's a bit extreme, but your nervous system doesn't know the difference. Modern stressors are related to real stressors. They might be third cousins twice removed, but they're still related.

We often don't let go of the ongoing and daily stressors and remain on a partial or complete red alert for a long period of time, sometimes not returning to a relaxed, balanced state until we're asleep. If you can even fall asleep, that is, and aren't tossing and turning, replaying the day's stressors. Again, stress hormones likely remain present because they are in constant production due to the continued perception of a continuing stressor.

Because we can't get to the relaxation response we need, our blood pressure and heart rate stay higher than they should, causing blood to rush through the circulatory system faster and harder than normal. This causes stress on the small interior skin cells (endothelial cells) lining the blood vessels. They can become "leaky" and allow cholesterol and free radicals to accumulate in the vessel walls that can cause them to harden (atherosclerosis) and become dysfunctional (endothelial dysfunction). The arteries harden, which means your blood vessels can no longer expand to accommodate the extra blood flow the next time the fight-or-flight response is evoked. In fact, the dysfunction can cause muscles in the arteries to tighten instead of loosen in response to the need for more blood flow, making the problem even worse. If the blood vessels are hardened, brittle, spasming, and inflexible, they might rupture or become blocked so no blood can get through. The result? A heart attack or stroke. Please note that this is an oversimplified description of heart attacks and strokes; the details are far more complex.

Now we have another problem. Your doctor tells you that your high blood pressure is dangerous. That's serious! The awareness that you have high blood pressure is a stressor in itself. Now you don't need the boss yelling at you anymore. You have your own built-in stressor to keep you in this dangerous loop. And high blood pressure is just one example.

The Energy Component to Stress

There is increasing evidence that stress produces other subtler and more serious changes as well. As we've already discussed, some researchers now suspect that the body is surrounded and governed by an electromagnetic energy field that is directly connected to its physical and emotional state of health, the energy matrix. The presence of this electromagnetic energy field is a major idea in energy healing.

- The energy matrix is affected by stress and responds *faster* than the body does, making it the first line of defense.

- The energy matrix may give us clues to disease *before* the body does or, at times, might even cause symptoms to signal you for help.

- The energy matrix, when properly balanced, can accelerate the body's own healing system.

Here's a classic example of the energy matrix at work: A tree falls and traps a young child. The mother dashes up, lifts the tree with superhuman strength, and pulls the child to safety. Surely no amount of adrenaline or psychological stimulus (love or fear) can account for this unbelievable phenomenon. We could inject a whole lot of adrenaline into your body but it wouldn't produce super-human strength. You'd be pretty jumpy, though. What's very likely is that under stress the mother was able to tap into a vast reservoir of energy through her energy matrix.

Now consider how being chewed out by your boss affects the entire system that governs and maintains your health. And it's not just a purely emotional or physical effect. Depending on how threatened you feel, you can experience a partial or total disruption of the stability or integrity of your energy matrix.

Scary stuff, right? But here's the good news: as you'll see later in the book, the effect on your energy matrix can be short-circuited. You can stop an inappropriate triggering of the fight-or-flight response before it gets started. You can learn to become conscious and immune to the energy effects of verbal stressors. You can even learn to augment your strength by positively and consciously activating your energy matrix.

Something to Try

Try this simple muscle test to see the power of verbal stressors. Ask a friend to extend his arm out to the side, perfectly straight with the elbow locked, and resist as you push down with steady pressure. Note the degree of resistance. Now tell your friend something that might cause him stress—"You're dirty; you smell; you're incompetent"—and push down on his arm again. You'll probably notice that the muscle is weaker. That's because the energy field, which accounts for some portion of his physical strength, has been short-circuited. Now say something complimentary and push down again. You'll notice that the arm has regained its strength.

The Sequence of Stress

We now understand that the human body is composed of three separate yet interrelated systems: the physical, the psychological, and the energy matrix. Stress appears to affect these three systems in a particular sequence:

1. The stressor enters your energy matrix, perhaps without your even realizing it. It might just be a sense or feeling that there's danger nearby.

2. Next, stress activates the body-mind (which functions like a psychological computer).

3. If the body-mind defines the stressor as threatening, it automatically triggers the physiological system, which turns on the whole fight-or-flight response.

You then prepare to battle it out or get away as fast as possible, which puts an end to the confrontation. Once the stressor is dealt with, all three systems slowly begin to come back to normal.

The point to remember is that your energy matrix is your first line of defense. What do we mean by that? While all of this is going on, the energy matrix tries to send signals to get you to calm down and enter the relaxation response stage. For example, you might develop an itch on an acupuncture point related to your nervous system, alerting you to the need for treatment. If you could just calm yourself down, the itch would go away. But you don't know that, so you scratch it, tear the skin, get an infection, and need additional treatment.

If we knew how to read the energy matrix, we would know this was a signal that we need to center ourselves. And if we knew how to balance the energy matrix through breathing, centering, self-massage, exercise, and energy healing, then we could eliminate many of these signal symptoms and focus on the ones that really need the healing. You'll learn how to do just that in Part 3.

The Stress-Block Cycle

When the fight-or-flight response kicks in and you can't fight or run, and there is a continued perception of stress (either conscious or subconscious), your body keeps producing the fight-or-flight hormones. These newly added hormones block you from returning to a restful state, hence the term stress-block.

Here's the cycle part of it: as your body continues to make these hormones, they can cause any number of diseases that, in turn, cause you more stress. It's like the gift that keeps on giving; these hormones are the stressor that keeps on stressing.

This is the stress-block cycle, the never-ending story of stress in the twenty-first century. And unlike the fight-or-flight or the relaxation responses, this one is not natural or good.

The stress-block cycle goes like this: You've got excess stress hormones being made by your body because of all that unchecked stress. Your energy matrix tries to get you to calm down by giving you a warning, maybe a headache. Instead of listening, you take a pill to cover up the symptom, but you ignore the cause. The energy matrix tries again, by giving you another symptom. And you ignore it—again—and take another pill. As the symptoms get worse and worse, your general health is deteriorating, which causes you more stress. So now the energy matrix's primary defense mechanism—giving you symptoms to calm you down—is making the problem even worse. Obviously the compounded stress-related symptoms and diseases we're describing here won't happen all in one day. We're talking about a long-term process that, unfortunately, plagues so many of us in one way or another. But remember: all of this can be prevented if you short-circuit the fight-or-flight response when it first enters your energy matrix and is interpreted as stressful.

Deeper connections

You know the old saying about the straw that broke the camel's back? Well, one straw never broke a camel's back. It was a whole lot of them. If we could eliminate the large number of inappropriately evoked stress responses—imagined or perceived stressors—we could probably handle the real ones a whole lot better.

The stress-block cycle is serious, but it's also our entry into the most hopeful part of energy healing. If we can learn to read the energy matrix— or find a healer or teacher who knows how to help us—we can begin to rebalance it with greater integrity so it will self-heal more effectively.

The Ultimate Stress Management

What can we do about stress? If we're to function properly in our nonstop world we must find techniques that enable us to ...

- Short-circuit the effects that stressors have on our energy matrix.

- Change our perception of stress to neutralize the unnecessary evoking of the fight-or-flight response. Once we learn to re-think an event as nonstressful, the physical fight-or-flight cycle won't be evoked. The stressor may then actually become a healthy motivator for creative and constructive action.

- Break up previously formed stress-blocks to help prevent the onset of certain diseases, while at the same time speeding up the body's capacity to heal itself.

- Monitor the energy matrix, the first line of defense that will tell us when and where new blocks are forming before they reach the body. We can do this with an energy healer or (at least in part) by ourselves.

- Learn to use daily challenges in an effective way that enables us to free our creative energies and open up to new levels of awareness.

You'll learn techniques to address each of these in later chapters.

Essential Takeaways

- Stress is the single-greatest threat to our well-being today.

- The autonomic nervous system has two parts: the sympathetic part evokes the fight-or-flight response, while the parasympathetic part evokes the relaxation response.

- Just as stress affects the physical body, there's a parallel process that affects the energy matrix.

- Handled poorly, stress can have a rapid and devastating effect on the energy matrix. If we understand the energy matrix, however, we can utilize it to our benefit.

chapter 5

Energy Healing
in Real Life

Conventional healing or energy healing?

Placebos, research, and biofeedback in energy healing

The difference between faith healing and energy healing

Making the choice to believe or disbelieve

We've almost reached the point of no return. We've established a common vocabulary, explored some ancient healing systems, dabbled in modern physics, and talked about the mind's power over the body. That's some pretty heavy stuff! But before we move forward, I want to take a moment to get real. In the many years I've spent healing and teaching, there have been certain questions, concerns, and reservations that have kept coming up, some of which have probably already occurred to you.

As we finish laying our foundation for the study of energy healing, let's cover some of the basics I think every student and practitioner should be familiar with.

What You Really Need to Know

Different systems of energy healing make different kinds of demands on the patient. Some systems ask nothing of a patient but to lie down on the table and receive the healing energy. Others give them remedies or "homework" practices they have to do on their own, some of which can be quite time consuming. I personally tend toward the latter approach because I find healing to be most effective when both the healer and the patient are engaged in the process, but both approaches can be highly effective.

If you're training to be an energy healer, obviously more work and depth is required. Here, too, some systems are heavier on the academic side of the training and some far less. Training might range from a few days to a few years. Without question, both approaches have proven track records of success and have produced highly competent healers.

When I train healers in my own system, called EnerGenesis, I lean toward a balance of academic and experiential. I teach a synthesis of basic anatomy and physiology, meridians, chakras, and sefirot. Students learn how to breathe, ground themselves, and do ocular divergence (see chapters 13–15). They learn complex maps for massage: for both themselves and the patients they see. Some of this training is for them to develop and upgrade their own energy matrix and some of it is to learn how to phase-lock with the patient. Most significantly, we explore the paradigm of a multi-dimensional WEB within which energy healing takes place. This is serious long-term training.

Do you need to know all of that to be a healer? Absolutely not. Many effective energy healers—my first teacher included—don't have that background. I personally like to engage my cognitive side as well as my more creative, intuitive side, but you can experience the phenomenon of energy healing, and learn to do it, without necessarily understanding it in detail.

However, having a broader perspective, one that encompasses some historical and scientific understanding, may enable the healer and the patient, in this data-filled world, to engage in the process more deeply. Maybe by exploring some of these early scientific attempts at explaining energy healing, you can better suspend your disbelief long enough to be helped.

Deeper Connections

When you interview your new baby's pediatrician, you probably want to know more than just where he went to medical school. If you feel strongly about a particular theory, you want to know that your doctor shares your commitment and perspective. Such is the case with energy healing; you don't need to be a master of every system, but you should know enough to ask the right questions.

Alternative, Complementary, and Conventional Medicine

One of the most common mistakes newcomers make is thinking they have to make a choice between energy healing and conventional medicine. That's absolutely not true. Often, the two can work very well together.

Language is often very telling. Alternative medicine, one of the terms used to describe different systems of energy healing, gives the impression that you can only do one or the other but not both. I think a better term is complementary medicine. Complementary leaves you with the feeling that the two can work together, complementing each other. When I see that something's out of balance—maybe I'm getting sick or having symptoms—I begin working on myself immediately with the skills I have. I also go to the doctor to find out what she believes the problem is. If it's something she can treat easily, I may take that medication while continuing to bolster my immune system with complementary techniques. For example, if I know that the antibiotic I'm taking is going to kill certain bacteria that I'll need for digestion, I might eat particular foods that will restore my balance. If my doctor can help point to the source of the problem, I can then do my part to help out the situation by working on the energy component.

The bottom line is that I don't rely on either system exclusively. Each modality has things that it does better and others it doesn't do as well. We've all heard similar stories from both sides.

Years ago, I knew of a patient who wasn't interested in being cured by energy healing. A biochemist who had a very scientific way of looking at the world, she was a close friend of my yoga and healing teacher, Greta. The woman had seen Greta do some pretty miraculous healings over the years, so when she developed cancer, she wanted to see if Greta could help bring up her white cell count high enough so she could tolerate chemotherapy. After the energy healing, the biochemist's blood count improved and she had the chemo treatments and was cured. I'd like to think she became a little more whole, too, as part of the process. In this case, the two worlds worked together beautifully. Another story comes to mind when the two worlds didn't work together so nicely. Years ago I was teaching a seminar at the Bowman Grey School of Medicine at Wake Forest University. One of the open-minded professors there had had some good personal results from our energy healing sessions together and wanted the third- and fourth-year medical students to open their minds a little and be exposed to this world.

But because I wasn't an MD, the department had a problem. They didn't want to call the seminar "Alternative Medicine" because I wasn't a physician; they seemed to think physicians held the copyright on the word medicine. In the end, we called it "Alternative Modalities in Family Care Practice," which was a decent compromise because it didn't make sense to anyone. Clearly, words make a difference. (Some of the amazing things that transpired from those lectures will be detailed in Chapter 16.)

The Placebo Effect

Skeptics often ask me whether energy healing is "just a placebo." Placebos are used as a control when new drugs or therapies are tested. Very generally, there's an expectation that up to 30 percent of the people in the control group (the ones taking the placebo, not the medication) will improve. The effectiveness of the drug is determined by a statistical comparison of the control group with the one getting the real drugs. If a placebo and the drug have the same success rate, then the drug isn't considered effective.

A Matter of Perspective

MISC.

A psychologist colleague of mine once told me this: among people who undergo classical Freudian psychotherapy, one third get better, one third stay the same, and one third get worse. However, among those who have no psychotherapy, a third get better, a third stay the same, and a third get worse. And he was a Freudian therapist!

Let's take a moment and look at what the placebo effect tells us. The body knows how to heal itself most of the time. Sometimes it needs a little help, a jumpstart from some form of chemical intervention. You take a drug and it prompts the body's immune system to act. It kills the invading bacteria and you get better.

But what makes the placebo work? We've already shown that in energy healing, the healer's thoughts can direct energy that triggers some action within the patient that trickles down to the body. Well, your thoughts are energy, too. Your own positive thought can trigger a positive effect on your energy matrix, which trickles down and affects your body. That doesn't mean the recovery is psychological, just that a change in thought can prompt a change in energy.

stay Grounded

Thinking positively is a good thing that sometimes can encourage the body to heal itself. But it doesn't always work because none of us (or very few, anyway) has an absolute and unequivocal control of our own mind all the time. We have doubts; we vacillate; we don't see results fast enough and wonder if we shouldn't have gone to the doctor earlier. These more negative thoughts have an effect on our energy matrix, too.

When people call energy healing a placebo, their key argument is that they went to an energy healer and felt better, but the problem came back. We learned earlier that healing is about finding the source of the energy blockage. In a case where the symptoms return, the healing may have moved some of the energy along the channel for a while, but the real block hadn't been uncovered yet.

The exact same thing happens when you take a pill that masks symptoms but doesn't find the source of the problem. When you stop taking the pill, the symptoms come back. One thing I can say about most energy healing is that it doesn't mask symptoms for any length of time. If it works, it works. If not, the symptoms will come back pretty quickly. But you won't be any worse off unless you avoided getting conventional medical input for too long and missed something really important. That's why I like to go to the doctor to get his or her input, too.

Scientific Research in Energy Healing

We talked about some of the advanced scientific theory behind energy healing, but if you're seriously thinking of going down this path, you may be wondering how much research there is to back it up … aside from the crazy things Puharich discovered in his basement, I mean!

There's a lot more going on out there than you might think. The National Institute of Health developed a whole branch to undertake high-quality, peer-reviewed research, and the website for the National Center for Complementary and Alternative Medicine has a wealth of information of systems research. You can find links to video sessions of some modalities, such as Reiki and acupuncture, and also look at sections earmarked for health professionals that highlight more serious research.

Why isn't there more? It's because of the research establishment. Ever wonder why there isn't more money for solar research, when we will inevitably need functional and affordable and renewable energy sources sooner rather than later? It doesn't make sense to me, either. The problem is that if you spend a lot of money on studies on energy healing and holistic therapies, you may not have anything to show for it—meaning a way to make your money back—when it's all over. Pharmaceutical companies spend a fortune on research but make it back selling the drugs that are approved. Sorry, folks, but there's no big money in the laying on of hands.

Actually, many areas of energy healing were part of early medical science until a number of systems related to the "body-electric" were removed from the curricula in the 1930s by the pharmaceutical companies that supported the medical schools.

To be fair, many of them should have been removed; in the early twentieth century, there was a lot of medical quackery around. At that time, electricity and radium were new. When the "radium girls," as they were called by the press, developed all sorts of diseases from painting watch dials by hand to get them to glow at night and then licked the brushes to get a good point for the next watch dial, no one could believe that the cause of the disease was the radium. It was the wonder drug; people all over the United States were drinking radium elixirs for energy and self-healing.

The Start of OSHA

OSHA, the Occupational Safety and Health Administration, is the main federal agency charged with the enforcement of safety and health regulations at work. Many of its regulations trace their origins back to the 1920s and the findings from the radium girls' cases.

Research is important. Just because something has been around for a few hundred—or a few thousand—years doesn't mean it can't be improved. Be sure to ask any prospective healer you approach if he can supply some sources of research in his modality.

The same thing is true of modern science. Methods for diagnosis and treatment that have been around for decades are constantly improving. When my mother-in-law was treated for cancer back in the late 1960s, the level of radiation was substantial. She was cancer-free for seven years, usually considered an all-clear sign, but she ultimately relapsed and died. When my sister-in-law was treated for the same disease 40 years later, she and her doctor discussed her mother's case. He pointed out that the dose of radiation used for their kind of tumor is much lower nowadays. The doctor felt it was probably the radiation that caused the recurrence that ultimately killed her mother; had she been diagnosed and treated today, she probably would have survived.

Just because there isn't a lot of research on a particular therapy doesn't mean it won't work. And don't assume the opposite, either, that if there *is* a lot of data, it's guaranteed to work. Just take it all with a grain of salt, and do your best to be an educated consumer.

Biofeedback Machines

Some of my students have used biofeedback machines to help them learn to enter a relaxed, meditative state. These devices don't actually relax or heal you themselves; they inform you of your state of mind by measuring and signaling changes in galvanic skin response, brain wave frequency, or through some other objective biological marker so you know when you're relaxed.

You're wired to a machine that beeps or blinks when a change is detected. That signal is an instantaneous feedback loop so you know that whatever you're doing is working. It might be breathing, mantra meditation, or some other technique. Usually the training is given over a five-to-six-week period, one session a week. Biofeedback machines can be great tools to help people learn how to reach an altered state of consciousness. The problem I've encountered with them is that when the patients no longer have the machines, they don't trust themselves to determine whether they're relaxed. That can lead to eventually abandoning the practice.

I can't tell you how many hundreds of times I've gone through the following dialogue:

> "Have you ever learned any stress-management skills?"
>
> "Yes. I studied biofeedback."
>
> "Good! How did it work?"
>
> "Terrific!"
>
> "Do you still practice the technique?"
>
> "Well, I did for a few months and then I stopped."
>
> "Why'd you stop?"
>
> "Well, I didn't have the machine, and …"

I prefer utilizing a built-in form of biofeedback. When you're doing cardiovascular exercise and you take your pulse to see if you've reached your target heart rate, that's biofeedback, too. It's using your biological systems to give you feedback on your current state without the machines.

When I teach breathing and rooting as a skill, I add a simple *Qi Gung* exercise. The feedback comes from the feel of the energy in and around your hands. True, it's subjective, but you don't need to plug into anything except the earth when you're rooting. (See Chapter 14 for more information on rooting.)

Qi Gung (or Chi Kung, Chi Gung, or Qi Gong, depending on whether you're speaking Mandarin or Cantonese) means energy exercise or energy discipline. *Kung Fu* (the same word Gung) means hard work and practice or discipline. And Kung Fu doesn't necessarily refer to a martial arts system. A master calligrapher, painter, or flower arranger could also be said to be doing Kung Fu.

Once you learn how to relax or meditate without machines, it can be fun to periodically see how you're doing with a more objective measurement device. The experiment I did at Clemson University (explained in Chapter 3) was a hoot. But I'd rather learn how to do these techniques without aids and then test them when I'm done. That way I'm never dependent on the machine.

Energy Healing and Faith Healing

During the time I spent in South Carolina when I talked about healing, I was often asked whether I meant faith healing. "Aren't energy healing and faith healing really the same thing?" The answer is no—and also yes. Let me explain.

As we've said before, there's one energy matrix, there's one WEB, and there's one energy, manifesting on many frequencies and going by many names. When looked at from that perspective, an energy healer and a bona fide faith healer are using the same energy.

Energy healing, however, leaves the faith of the individual out of the equation. Individual healers and patients can have their own very different spiritual or religious paradigms. In the Kabbalistic model presented in Chapter 2, for example, we referred to the Ayn-Sof as the Infinite One. It probably comes as no surprise that the Kabbalists believe this to be God. You don't have to agree or disagree; the more open-minded you are, the more likely you are to benefit from energy healing and/or become a successful energy healer.

Just as the healer's mind has to be in an altered state of readiness to engage in the healing process, so the patient's mind has to be open to receiving the energy. For some people, the only way to enter that state is to use words like faith or God in their healing. For others, the words aren't necessary. Let each march to the beat of his or her own paradigm.

There was a film years ago called *Resurrection* starring Ellen Burstyn and Sam Shepard. Burstyn played a woman who has a near-death experience. When she awakens from a coma, she possesses the miraculous gift of being able to heal others. After she helps to facilitate some major unexplainable cures, she reluctantly agrees to let science study her abilities. Her old boyfriend, however, doesn't like to see this kind of energy healing without a little religion thrown in. He fears that if you don't mention God, the healing must come from a darker, evil source.

The key point here is that all the energy in the universe, whether of a higher vibration or a lower frequency, comes from the same place. It's neither good nor evil. It's the intention of the user that alters the energy. Open your mind to that idea and don't get caught up in the words.

Considering words, these may offer some perspective. Chuang Tzu, an ancient Taoist Master, wrote:

> The fish trap exists to catch the fish; when you've caught the fish, you no longer need the trap.
>
> The bird snare exists to catch the bird. When you've got the bird in hand, you no longer need the snare.
>
> Words exist to get the meaning. When you have the meaning, you no longer need the words.
>
> Where can I find a man who has forgotten all the words, so I can have a word with him?

Believing and Disbelieving

One of the most commonly asked questions about energy healing is also, in my opinion, one of the most important: do you have to believe in energy healing for it to work?

The simple answer is no. Your personal beliefs don't affect the existence of energy—or energy healing—one way or the other. It's not like that famous scene in *Peter Pan* when the only way to bring Tinker Bell back to life is to say you believe in fairies.

The truth is, what you believe doesn't alter the composition of the physical world. People used to believe the world was flat, but that didn't contribute to a single incident of anyone falling off the edge … at least not that I know of. On the other hand, just because you can't see oxygen doesn't mean you have to believe in it in order to breathe.

Here's the key: even if you're not a believer, I encourage you to try not to be a zealous disbeliever. Think back to the water crystals we dealt with in Chapter 3, and how thoughts and words affected them. The energy of your thoughts is real. If you're sitting with an energy healer thinking energy healing is all a bunch of baloney, you could negatively affect her ability to send positive energy. That will make the session unsuccessful, which will strengthen your belief that it's nonsense. It's a vicious cycle of negativity.

It's similar to acoustics, the science of sound. You can have two sound waves playing at the same time. Depending on their frequency, they can amplify the final sound (by creating constructive interference patterns) or one can cancel out the other (destructive interference patterns). Think of the constructive sound waves as positive thoughts and the destructive sound waves as negative ones.

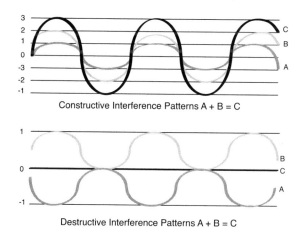

Constructive and destructive interference patterns.

It's possible that negative thought energy could interfere with whatever healing energy is at work. So you don't have to believe in energy healing, necessarily, but it helps if you don't vigorously disbelieve it. Suspend your disbelief and you never know what you'll discover.

Essential Takeaways

- You don't have to be an expert on every aspect of energy healing to benefit from it; just try to keep an open mind.

- A choice to pursue energy healing shouldn't replace conventional medicine; the two worlds are complementary.

- While energy healing isn't just a placebo, positive thoughts can trigger a change in your energy matrix that can kick-start recovery.

- There's research to support energy healing, but not nearly enough, and some of it should be taken with a grain of salt.

- Biofeedback machines and other measuring devices can be a fun way to test your progress, but don't rely on them too heavily.

- Faith healing is similar to energy healing in that both try to tap into a higher energy, but energy healing does so while leaving faith and religion out of the equation.

- You don't have to believe in energy healing for it to work, but try not to actively disbelieve it; negative thoughts can interfere with healing.

Part 2

Energy Healing Systems

There are a multitude of energy healing systems out there, utilizing many strategies and techniques. We're going to take a sampling of them to give you an overview. By the time we're done, you'll be able to categorize and understand virtually any healing system you encounter.

First, we'll explore a broad variety of diagnostic approaches, many of which are used in every system out there, albeit in different combinations and with different emphasis.

Then we'll look at different types of healing systems that may seem very different, but as we look a little more closely, we'll see that they all rely on the healer entering into a specific state of consciousness and attitude for healing. These categories include systems that use laying on of hands or soft-touch energy modalities, massage, and tools that facilitate healing, including water, crystals, needles, pendulums, herbs … even music and diet!

Finally, we'll touch briefly on the subject of remote-view healing, where the healer is in a different location from the patient, sometimes even on the other side of the world!

chapter 6

Methods of Diagnosis in Energy Healing

Exploring methods of energy diagnosis

Reading the holographic energy matrix

Elevated sight, hearing, and touch

Whether you're an energy healer or a conventional doctor, the first step is the same: you have to find out what's wrong with a patient before you can treat him. There are many different diagnostic methods used in energy healing, but the goal is always to phase-lock with the patient's energy matrix to find the blockages, excesses, or deficiencies of energy. The internal systems (blood, organs, nervous system, skeletal structure, etc.) give off subtle external signs that can be read, but it takes a fair amount of time to master.

Chinese Pulse Diagnosis

When you go to a conventional doctor, one of the first things she does is check your pulse, or heart rate. Well, if you go to a t'ai chi healer, he'll check the same thing, but he isn't feeling/sensing for the same information. An acupuncturist, for example, as one type of t'ai chi healer, relies on the pulses to give primary information on the state of the 12 meridians.

Remember, we're using the term t'ai chi healing as the overall umbrella term to refer to any system whose foundation is built on the t'ai chi, the supreme ultimate principle of yin and yang.

On each wrist there are three positions, each of which are pressed two ways, deeply and lightly, for a total of six positions. These positions provide the healer with the status of your meridians. The deeper position is for the ones that are yin, and the shallow or superficial position is for the ones that are yang. This follows the same pairing of organs that's used for the body's circulation of energy: each yin organ has a corresponding yang organ.

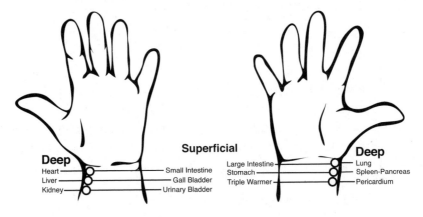

Chinese pulse relationships.

In his classic work *Acupuncture: The Ancient Chinese Art of Healing and How It Works Scientifically*, Dr. Felix Mann lists the 28 qualities most commonly felt for in pulse diagnosis. There are many more, and with all these variations, stories persist of incredible expertise in the hands of a master of acupuncture.

A colleague once witnessed an incredible experiment where such a master attempted to diagnose a patient using nothing but those six positions. They didn't speak beforehand, nor did the acupuncturist see the patient, who put his hands through two holes cut in a white sheet so his facial expressions couldn't be read. After feeling/listening to the pulse, with all its subtleties and variations, for a few minutes, the acupuncturist was not only able to offer an accurate diagnosis but also provide a complete medical history, including every major illness the patient ever had, how long ago it was, and whether there were any residual energy blocks that needed to be dealt with. These masters would probably put TV's Dr. House to shame with their uncanny diagnostic abilities.

The three pulse positions also represent top-to-bottom and inside-to-outside correspondences. With all three fingers in the correct positions, the acupuncturist asks the body about general levels of energy from the top of the head to the diaphragm (Position 1), from the diaphragm to the Tan T'ien, or lower center of gravity (Position 2), and from the Tan T'ien to the bottom of the feet (Position 3).

Next, with his fingers in the same positions, he asks the body about the nature of the energy from the outer perimeter of the body moving inward: outer (skin and muscles), middle (organs and nerves), and inner (bones).

It's important to note that there are many variations in pulse diagnosis, and not every system agrees on which meridian is connected to which pulse position. If one healer believes the third pulse position tells us that the kidney meridian is weak and another thinks that position is related to the heart meridian, can they both be right? How can different healers utilize variations of a particular modality and still get correct results?

Deeper connections	In an exhaustive treatise on *The Pulse in Occident and Orient, Its Philosophy and Practice in Holistic Diagnosis and Treatment,* Amber and Babey-Brooke present four differing major Chinese systems alone. In addition, they outline Chinese variations and present differing systems of pulse taking from Western, ancient Greek, Ayurvedic, and Arabic sources.

You have to remember that the healer isn't simply interested in pulses to get information about blood running through an artery. Feeling the different qualities of the pulses requires a much subtler level of perception. In an altered state, the healer phase-locks with the patient's energy matrix, mentally asks the questions, and waits for the answer. Each healer operates within his own pulse paradigm; what he asks for is what he gets.

While it might seem confusing, pulse-taking is actually an incredibly flexible system because it relies heavily on the healer's state of consciousness. Using the pulses, the energy matrix can provide any and all information. He just has to know how to ask.

Japanese Facial Diagnosis

You may be familiar with the idea of the micro-expressions that are featured on certain television shows or in films. The trained practitioner, usually working with the police or an intelligence agency, looks at someone and, like a human lie detector, can tell whether he's hiding something or suppressing some deeper level of emotion. This is accomplished by noting incredibly subtle movements and expressions on the face. There are over 3,000 such micro-expressions, and experts in this area are few.

The underlying premise in using these expressions for energy diagnosis is that each individual's outside represents a visible, living history of its inside condition, history, and development. If you have the skills to understand and read it, you can derive an accurate history and diagnosis of the patient's energy matrix.

In facial diagnosis, subtle variations are sought from the patient's face, but here they relate to underlying energy disturbances. Look at the chart below. Notice that the upper lip is related to the energy condition of the stomach. The lower lip relates to the condition of the intestines. The kidneys are seen in the recesses under your eyes.

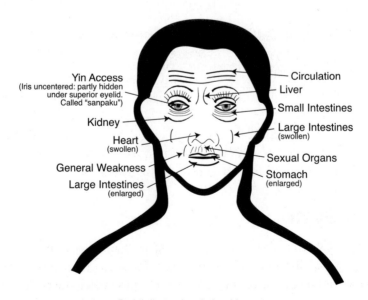

Facial diagnosis relationships.

Clearly, we all have those body parts, and the condition of the color, lines, swelling, etc., of the face may show that everything is normal inside. Or it may show that something is out of balance.

With centuries of cases, and massive amounts of data collected both formally and informally from around the world, certain relationships between the meridians and the face have been observed and confirmed. These connections enable the diagnostician to assess the condition of the meridians beneath the surface.

Before you run to a mirror and freak out at every blemish, I suggest you relax a bit. It's probably just a mark on your face and not a deep, diagnostic discovery. You might feel that way when your dentist shows you an X-ray of your teeth. He says, "See that spot? That's a cavity." But then you ask about another spot that looks exactly the same and he replies, "Oh, that's nothing." Always raise the question, but trust a skilled energy diagnostician to determine when there really is a problem.

There are many other diagnostic maps that provide as much detail as the face does. The face, of course, includes the eyes, ears, mouth, and hair. The skin is also a major source of information. The hands include the pulses, the lines on the palms, and the nails. The voice, handwriting, gait, diet, gestures, and habits may all be sending messages that are used to diagnose your energy matrix, which includes your energy organs and psycho-emotional states as well. Each of these areas contains whole databases of information on the overall energy balance of the patient.

It may be a little humbling to realize how much of your overall well-being is an open book to those who know how to read it. As a patient, don't get paranoid about your privacy being invaded; very few people can do this kind of reading, nor would they do it without your permission. Remember, a healer must be invited to read someone's energy matrix.

Micro-Systems

In the early 1950s, the French acupuncturist Dr. Paul Nogier made a groundbreaking discovery. When looking at the ancient charts of acupuncture points on the ear, he connected the dots and saw that the placement of the points was perfectly logical when placed over a diagram of a human fetus.

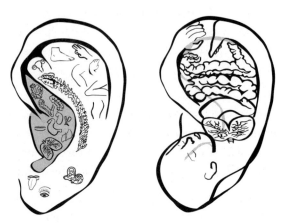

Auricular therapy and fetus correspondence.

Until that point (pardon the acu pun), acupuncture points followed the meridians; Nogier discovered that points relating to the entire body could be found on the ear.

Twenty years later, Dr. Ralph Alan Dale, an acupuncturist and scholar, furthered Nogier's work by looking at other areas—the hands, the feet, even the eyes—and discovering that numerous systems exist all over the body. Dr. Dale coined the term micro-acupuncture, referring to any system where one part of the body manifests reflexes to every main meridian and organ. He referred to the traditional meridians and points distributed all over the body as macro-acupuncture.

stay Grounded

The term micro-acupuncture doesn't necessarily mean that needles will be used. Because some of the 20-plus systems deal with small (and sometimes delicate) parts of the body, many of these systems use pressure, or even electricity, to stimulate the points. Other systems (like the eye, for example) are purely for diagnosis.

Holographic Access Systems

When they hear the term micro-acupuncture, most people think of needles. I prefer to use the term holographic access system because, like a hologram, each part of the energy matrix can be accessed through a smaller part of the whole.

To really understand this analogy, you need a very basic understanding of holograms. If you take a photograph of an apple and develop the negative, you'll get a picture of the apple. If you cut that negative into 20 little pieces and develop one of those pieces, you'd get a picture of just what was on that particular piece (presumably 1/20 of the apple).

By contrast, if you shine a laser through a holographic negative of an apple, the lasers will produce the image of a 3-D apple floating in space. If you cut that negative into 20 pieces and shine a laser through any of the pieces, you'd still see the whole apple! Each little piece has the whole apple in it.

The idea of the holographic access system is that each part of the energy matrix can be accessed through a smaller part of the whole. If we can graph the liver on the hands or ears or feet, we can palpate that point on the holographic access system and affect the liver and its related meridians.

Auricular-Therapy

In order to use the holographic access system of the ear for diagnosis, we would have to use pressure on a particular point with a small probe. If the point is tender, a problem is indicated. Many contemporary auricular-therapists prefer to do this form of diagnosis with electronic equipment because the area is so small, and relying on the patient's reaction is a little subjective.

There's an electro-acupuncture device in which you set parameters for an acceptable level of current and touch the ear's acupoint with an electronic probe. If the current flowing through the contacted point is lower or higher than the set parameters, the machine emits a small beeping sound. The acupuncturist then knows that the point is a problem that needs to be treated.

Iridiagnosis

The holographic access system of the eye is referred to as iridiagnosis, or iridology. *Naturopaths* often use it as a diagnostic method and then follow up with treatments including diet, vitamins, minerals, supplements, and homeopathic remedies.

finding
Meaning
Naturopathy is a system of alternative medicine based on the principle of vitalism. Both MDs and non-MDs practice naturopathy. The treatment aspect focuses on natural self-healing: diet, lifestyle changes, and natural supplements. While some say the ideas go back to Hippocrates, most date the development of naturopathy to the nineteenth century European nature-cure movement.

While the discovery of modern iridiagnosis is generally credited to Von Peckzely in the nineteenth century, Phillipus Meyens did much earlier work in the seventeenth century. The principle remains the same as with all holographic access systems: every organ and body part is represented on a specific area on the iris, where changes in the health of the patient are reflected by certain signs, marks, and discolorations. By observing the changes in the eyes alone, the practitioner can derive the patient's tendencies toward health and disease and her general well-being, as well as the state of each individual organ.

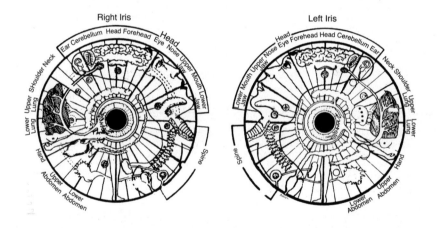

Iris diagnosis chart.

A competent iridologist can form a diagnosis this way with much success. Often, the iridologist will take photos of the iris and project them onto a screen. This way, details that might have escaped notice are clearly seen in the enlargement.

Clear Sensing and the Energy Matrix

You've probably heard the term clairvoyance before. Two other related terms—clairaudience and clairsentience—might not be as familiar. Essentially, these terms mean clear seeing, clear hearing, and clear feeling, or clear sensing, collectively. The word "clear" in this context means not limited by considerations of space or time. If you can enter a trance state and see someone or something miles away, beyond the range of your physical eyes—without Skype or iChat!—that experience would be clairvoyant. If you hear voices that aren't heard by anyone present, perhaps a spirit-guide or teacher from another plane of reality, that's clairaudience. Bluetooth voices and psychotic delusions don't count! And if you can sense something that's not in your physical environment (or reality), that's clairsentience. Scanning the energy matrix for energy healing fits into that category.

Many healers specialize in one of the three, although often they'll have developed basic skills and familiarity with the others as well.

Clairvoyance: Clear Seeing

When you think of an aura, you probably think of a colored halo-type energy field surrounding the human body that only some people can see. But if you think back to our definition of the energy matrix as the energy component of our physical bodies, seeing auras takes on a whole new perspective. Clairvoyants are those with the ability to see the human aura—or the energy matrix—with the naked eye.

On the following page is a simple illustration of a basic auric field as seen by a clairvoyant. The auric field is highly differentiated and complex, just as the human body is. Getting a sense of an aura from this illustration would be like getting a sense of the human nervous, circulatory, and digestive systems by looking at a family portrait; you're just going to see the surface! An experienced and accomplished clairvoyant can see things that novices won't. What they see depends somewhat on the inborn or developed mastery they possess of their own energy matrix, and somewhat on their training with a master of that skill.

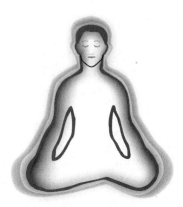

The human aura.

One of the most remarkable works in using clairvoyant skills for healing is Barbara Ann Brennan's *Hands of Light: A Guide to Healing Through the Human Energy Field*. She began her career as a research scientist for NASA and has spent years researching, practicing, and teaching energy healing. She's a highly gifted clairvoyant, seeing many things in the human aura that the novice can't.

Almost anyone can learn to see a very basic level of the human aura. Whether that evolves into a deeper mastery depends on the individual. Start by quieting the mind, and running through some of the techniques covered in Part 3 of this book. Once you know how to breathe and root, try gazing in the direction of your friend in ocular divergence, and allowing yourself to see more than what your eyes can see around his head. This may sound lofty and metaphorical, but with a little practice—and an open mind—you never know what you'll be able to see!

MISC.

Aura-Viewing Experiment

Once you think you can see auras, here's a fun experiment you can try at home. Cover your subject's face with a thin cloth, so you can't read her face. Once you can see her aura, have a third person read a list of 20 foods (prepared in advance). Ask the subject to think about how she feels about the foods. Based on what her aura does—brighten for positive feelings, diminish for negative—mark down how you think she feels, and then compare your results!

Years ago, a very fine clairvoyant and I decided to conduct an experiment in blind diagnosis: We would find someone neither of us had ever met, take no verbal history and each do our own form of energy diagnosis, recording exactly what we sensed. Then we would talk with the person to determine how correct we were, and how close we were to each other in our energy diagnoses.

One of my students brought in a stranger. The clairvoyant and I both went through our paces, she by viewing the subject's aura and I by scanning the energy matrix with my hands. Neither of us ever made physical contact with the person.

We both sensed congestion in the lungs, strain on the adrenals, and tension in the lower back. The woman later confirmed that she had asthma and lower-back pain. The interesting thing was how our diagnostic descriptions matched up. The clairvoyant saw cloudy, dark energy surrounding the lungs, while I felt thick, compacted energy in the same place. She saw flashing, reddish lesions on the lower back and I felt sharp, prickly agitated energy in the same place. She saw dull, tired colors around the adrenal glands and I felt low, exhausted, and deficient energy as I passed the adrenals. We matched up 100 percent—and, more important, we both found the primary energy blockages and imbalances in the woman.

Fortunately, the third and fourth chakras that were involved in this immune-related issue were relatively easy to help. In a few sessions her asthma was virtually gone, the back pain—which was probably a message from her energy matrix to deal with the asthma in the first place—had disappeared, and she began a daily breathing regimen that was deeper than any breath she had taken in years. It was a fun experiment and a successful healing.

As a final thought, there is a well-known phenomenon called the phantom-leaf effect. It was discovered that when a *Kirlian photograph* was taken of a leaf at set periods after it was torn, it seemed to show an energy aura where the missing portion of the leaf would have been. As the leaf withered, the aura diminished.

More related to healing, an experiment was conducted where a part of the limb of a limb-regenerating salamander was cut off. A Kirlian photograph showed the aura of the limb remained and, in time, the limb regenerated as expected. In a second version of the same experiment, an electrical probe was used to disperse and disrupt the energy field around the torn limb. This time, the limb failed to regenerate. This would indicate that the organizing field—or aura—that was photographed was necessary for the limb to regenerate.

Kirlian photography is a form of high-voltage photography named after Semyon Kirlian. In 1939, Kirlian accidentally discovered that if you run 20,000 volts across a photographic plate to pump it up, when the photons drop out of orbit, they emit a light that can be recorded on a photographic plate. Kirlian said that the image he was studying might be compared with the human aura.

Many people ask if Kirlian photography can actually photograph an aura. Think of the image as a shadow of the energy field, not the energy field itself. This shadow is visible in the photograph because it was pumped up with electricity. It's like a pencil-rub drawing; if you take a piece of paper, put a penny underneath it, and rub the pencil over it, it will create an image of the coin, but it's not the same as a photograph of the penny. It's only a shadow of the original. Still, the picture is remarkable and can help you to visualize what an aura might look like.

Clairaudience: Clear Hearing

Expert clairaudients are much rarer than clairvoyants. One exceptional clairaudient was Arigo, the "surgeon with a rusty knife" from Brazil. Until his death in the early 1970s, he healed thousands of patients with energy healing and psychic surgery. His work had been documented on film by a team of physicians headed by Dr. Puharich.

In the film, Arigo takes a kitchen paring knife, inserts it under the lid of the eye of a patient, and scrapes off the cataract forming on the eye. This was done without any kind of anesthesia, yet there was no pain reported by the patient. Moreover—and this may be the most amazing part of what he did—the patient was able to see without the implant of an artificial lens to replace what was removed by the knife. There was no bleeding and no infection!

Eye surgeons have watched this video in complete and utter shock. But here's the craziest part: One day, as Puharich was watching him do this procedure, Arigo placed the knife in Puharich's hand and proceeded to do the surgery, guiding his hand throughout. Puharich described the sensation as if a force-field was surrounding the knife so it couldn't move anywhere but where the field allowed it. It was like a sheath of energy, so the knife could do no harm to the patient as long as Arigo was holding his hand. He said it was one of the most amazing things he ever felt.

Arigo only had an elementary school education, and when asked how he was able to do the incredible things he did—from surgery to writing prescriptions after just looking at a patient for a few seconds—he replied that he heard the voice of a Dr. Fritz talking to him in his left ear, inside his head, telling him what to do. He always did exactly as he was told, and his success rate was off the charts.

Did We Pass?

MISC.

When Arigo was asked why he thought he had been blessed with these amazing abilities, his answer was, "I'm here to take the temperature of the human race!" That might seem like a relatively innocuous statement, but when coming from a man like Arigo, it makes you wonder. He was here on Earth, but from where? What was the test? And if he was testing the human race to see if it's ready to expand our global paradigm, did we pass?

Clairsentience: Clear Feeling

Clairsentience in the world of energy healing, just like clairvoyance and clairaudience, consists of being attuned to your energy matrix and then phase-locking with the patient's energy matrix. Once phase-locked, you scan the energy matrix and download diagnostic information from it, preparing you to begin the healing or uploading of healing intent. Anyone can be trained to do this at some level with techniques of breathing, centering, and ocular divergence. Many of the basics will be covered in Part 3 of this book.

In addition to scanning with your hands, clairsentience refers to the internal process when you have a feeling about something. It could be an emotional response or something more specific: "I feel you should skip that airplane flight and catch the next one." We've all heard stories about that sort of premonition surfacing on September 11, 2001.

The key seems to be asking the correct yes-or-no questions and then quieting the mind enough to sense the response. But you have to know the difference between your own imagination and a message from a higher reality, or to put it more poetically, know the sound of your own music. You have a sense within you that whatever thought or feeling you just had is worth paying attention to, that it's not just reverie but a response to your silently asked question.

If a thought pops into your head, it doesn't mean it came from heaven, a spirit guide, an angel, or an extraterrestrial. It may just be your imagination improvising. Whatever information you get in an altered state should be scrutinized and tested, when possible, before you sell your house and begin a year-long retreat in the Himalayas. Try not to lose sight of the fact that you could be wrong.

As subjective as this all sounds, it's a real ability that can be developed with the aid of a teacher. The training, however, should be done with caution and care.

Essential Takeaways

- Many diagnostic systems are based on reading the physiognomy of the body, including diagnosis by reading the face, tongue, eyes, feet, hands, and so forth.

- One can be trained to read the many maps that exist on the surface of the body to diagnose internal energy imbalances.

- Think of the energy matrix as a hologram, where every part has access to all the information of the whole.

- A large number of diagnostic systems are holographic access systems from which we can download information about the well-being of the energy matrix.

- We can learn to expand and heighten our abilities to see, hear, and touch the energy matrix to gather information.

chapter 7

Energy Healing Treatments Through Laying On of Hands

Ancient healing methods

Three modern systems

Scientific methods and results

Laying on of hands is one of the most common modalities of energy healing. You might even be familiar with stories about laying on of hands; early biblical and other references to prophets, shamans, and medicine men and women often feature a version of the practice. What the stories have in common is that someone comes to a healer with a problem, who then puts his or her hands on them or above them and attempts to pass some kind of divinely channeled healing light through to the patient.

Let's look at some of the systems to give you a "feel" for what's out there.

Qi Gung

While the words Qi Gung are Chinese, you can find some version of this energy healing exercise in almost every ancient culture on the planet. It's not just a technique done by a healer; it's a meditation exercise that anyone can practice to evoke self-healing, or to complement what a teacher/healer might be doing.

Let's look at two of the most famous Qi Gung exercises as examples, known today as the microcosmic orbit and the macrocosmic orbit. Both meditative exercises focus on guiding the energy flow through the channels of the energy matrix. This is an essential part of the training of a healer, since it simultaneously grounds the healer and upgrades the energy he or she channels.

 You wouldn't stick a screwdriver into an electrical outlet without being properly grounded. Similarly, there are a few pre-requisites to help ground you so you can practice Qi Gung safely and successfully. You have to be able to enter an alpha/theta-range meditative state (7–8 hz). You have to root to the earth (see Chapter 14), or phase-lock with the 8 hz heartbeat of the planet. And it helps to know the exact pathway within your body through which you want to move the energy.

As with many Qi Gung exercises, you begin microcosmic orbit meditation with breathing techniques to quiet and focus the mind. Bring your attention to the tan t'ien, the lower center of your energy matrix, your physical center of gravity and the point below and behind your navel from which you generate your deep breathing (see Chapter 13).

You would then guide the energy with your mind, from your lower center downward to the base of your spine and upward through your spinal energy channels. Let it flow over the top of your head and down the front of your body (following specific meridians), and when it reaches the base of your spine again the energy goes back to the lower center. This cycle is repeated a number of times. The process is designed to cleanse your energy channels and upgrade your energy capacity.

The macrocosmic orbit begins the same way, but extends the torso orbit by continuing the energy journey out through the arms and legs and, in some versions, even down to the center of the earth. Even with these simple orbits, there are many variations, so if you've learned a technique that's slightly different, practice it the way you've been taught.

Deeper connections

Every Asian system has a word for the navel center. What is called dantian (dan t'ian, dan tien, or tan t'ien) in China and Thailand is called tanden in Japan and danjeon in Korea.

Japanese systems use the term tanden interchangeably with the term hara. In the Japanese tradition, a master of calligraphy, swordsmanship, tea ceremony, or martial arts is said to be "acting from the hara." Whatever the language or system, this energy center is an important focal point in many internal meditative techniques.

In many techniques of Qi Gung, you will also find slow-motion movements of the hands, drawing them up and down or over the head or out to the side. Each of these movements has the same goal in mind: to move energy around the energy matrix through the various channels, meridians, etc. One simple exercise is explained in Chapter 14.

Kabbalistic Laying On of Hands

The *Sefer Yetzirah: The Book of Creation*s is one of the oldest and most mysterious of all Kabbalistic texts in the Jewish tradition. References to the book go back as far as the first century of the Common Era, and traditions regard the work as originally an oral transmission from biblical days, well over 1,000 years earlier.

The late Rabbi Aryeh Kaplan, a highly regarded authority and scholar, wrote a contemporary commentary on the work in which he states something extraordinary about the tree of life, the sefirot, and the laying on of hands for spiritual healing.

Misc.

A Mystic and Scholar

There is probably no greater modern scholar on the theory and practice of Jewish meditation than Rabbi Aryeh Kaplan. Drawn from his intimate knowledge of both science and Kabbalah, his well-documented books have inspired a generation of Jewish meditators and healers to look within their own roots for guidance and direction in this very esoteric arena. His death in his early 50s was a terrible loss.

Kaplan explains that normally the 10 sefirot are shown in the three columns you saw in the diagram of the tree of life in Chapter 2. When they're in that form, they're at rest. The male column on the right and the female column on the left are each kept in a stable state of equilibrium by the central column. But what happens when that central column takes sides, dividing its sefirot to the right or left?

When the sefirot are drawn in two columns, five sefirot each, they take on a male/female (or yin/yang) polarity of spiritual tension. In that polarized formation, they become very powerful and can be utilized for deepened prayer or healing or blessing others.

The *Sefer Yetzirah* links the 10 sefirot to the 10 fingers. When the hands are together, the energies are stable. But when the mystic, healer, or prayer wants to direct these powerful energies, he separates the hands and polarizes the sefirot. If you think about it, it's actually quite similar to water: H_2O. In its normal state, water is stable and balanced, but if you separate the hydrogen and oxygen, these two elements are highly volatile. Hydrogen fuel cells in the presence of oxygen power the craft we send into space. And that same hydrogen atom from stable H_2O can also produce the hydrogen bomb!

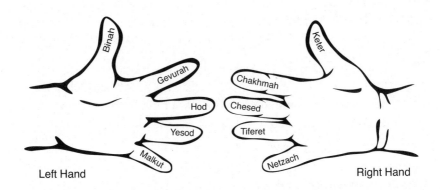

Kabbalistic Hands From Sefer Yetzirah

Kabbalistic hands with sefirot.

Once the sefirot are polarized, they can then be channeled and focused through the consciousness of the healer through the hands to achieve the desired effect. All of this requires deep training in meditation, concentration, and *kavana*.

Finding Meaning

Kavana is a Hebrew word (from the root kē'vūn, aim or direction) that means directed consciousness, attention, or disciplined spiritual imagination. On a more practical level, it means concentration, focus, or intention. There's a famous saying in Hebrew: "Prayer without kavana is like a body without a soul." Most healing systems spend a great deal of time exploring the intention of the healer. (See Chapter 17.)

To this day, at special times during the Jewish year, the cohanim—the priestly caste, descendants of Moses' brother Aaron—bless the people of the congregation by raising their hands in a special configuration to channel these powerful spiritual forces.

You don't have to be Jewish to be familiar with the hand configuration of this ancient blessing. The famous Vulcan greeting in *Star Trek*—"Live long and prosper!"—is the exact hand position the cohanim use. Leonard Nimoy, the actor who played Mr. Spock, suggested using the hand position to the writers of the show. He had seen it as a child when his grandfather took him to an Orthodox synagogue and it left a strong impression on him.

Silva Mind Method

In more modern times, new systems of energy healing have developed that use the laying on of hands. One of the early popular systems in the West, the Silva Mind Method, is a technique to quiet and focus the mind and thereby develop skills of healing and clairvoyance.

Jose Silva, an electronics engineer, began his research on the human brain out of love for his 10 children. He wanted to help them do better in school. Silva found that brain cells functioned more effectively when the brain slowed down, when they became more open to receiving and storing information. In other words, the alpha brain wave was the place to begin deeper energy work. By 1966, he had developed the Silva Method, a personal development program that provides tools to enhance one's quality of life. So many of the discoveries Silva incorporated into his approach echo the energy paradigm you've been learning about. Here is a breakdown of his basic ideas:

- You begin by reaching a state of controlled relaxation to enhance the potential strengths of the mind.

- In that state of mind, you can trigger inspiration and creativity, heighten memory, accelerate learning, and harmonize your brain's hemispheres.

- Operating in the beta frequency of 15–30 hz helps you to think logically, sequentially, and analytically.

- Operating in the alpha dimension of 7–14 hz helps you to activate the right brain's strengths for rhythm, color appreciation, creative imagination, and intuition.

- Operating in alpha will also enable you to improve visualization, mental projection or remote viewing, and positive thinking.

Case studies speak of reduced stress levels, overcoming shyness and anxiety, and loss of headaches and symptoms of depression.

Deeper Connections

For centuries, techniques such as laying on of hands and remote viewing have been practiced in cultures around the world. Sometimes advanced skills were kept in the hands of the leaders, teachers, and healers of these civilizations to maintain some degree of control over the masses. The Silva Method helped publicize many of these techniques and brought them into the public forum of the modern era.

One of the techniques taught in Silva classes is psychometry—the ability to touch an object and pick up vibrations about its history, ownership, etc. In one sense, all energy healing involves a sort of psychometric process, as the healer must phase-lock with the patient's energy matrix and receive impressions from it.

Psychometry is often used in ESP research because it can be easily tested in a double-blind format. An object is given to a neutral third party and placed in a sealed package. The package is sent to the psychometrist, who holds it and then records any impression received, either with words or pictures. Meanwhile, the neutral party interviews the owner of the object and makes his or her own written account of the actual background and history of the object. Neither the psychometrist nor the owner of the object know each other or have any contact throughout the process. By comparing the two accounts, you can measure the accuracy of the psychometrist.

To give you an idea of how this works, a Silva graduate was given an old piece of jewelry. He closed his eyes and breathed quietly for a few minutes. Then he picked up the object and held it in his closed hand for three or four minutes. Then he wrote down what he sensed: a description of the owner, the house he lived in, how many children he had, and a few other bits of information. He was approximately 70 percent accurate, an impressive score.

The Silva Method is a very systematic way of entering into a grounded, centered state. Silva talks about the beat of the earth and its 7–8 hz heartbeat (the Schumann Resonance of 7.82 hz, mentioned earlier). Using our vocabulary, we might describe what they do as getting in touch with one's energy matrix and logging on to the WEB. Once in that state of mind, virtually everything that the Silva Method claims its graduates can do is not only possible but has been around for millennia in one culture or another. They seem to have a very organized and systematic way of accomplishing that result.

Reiki

Another very popular form of healing using the laying on of hands that has reached the West is called Reiki. Legend claims that Dr. Mikao Usui, a Japanese monk, gained the knowledge and spiritual power to apply and attune others to *Reiki*, which entered his body through the crown chakra, during a peak experience or mystical revelation in 1922.

Finding Meaning

Reiki is usually translated as universal life energy, but some say it derives from another Japanese word that means mysterious atmosphere. The syllable ki (in Chinese, qi or chi) means life force or breath, while rei translates as spirit, miraculous, or divine. Reiki is another on our list of words to define our intangible healing energy.

After Usui's death, Reiki went through a variety of changes. Today there are two major branches: traditional Japanese Reiki and Western Reiki. The traditional form seems to be more intuitive and the Western form more structured.

Reiki is generally instructed at three levels. The first level deals with basic healing abilities. The second level introduces remote healing, a deeper study of the flow of energy, and the use of symbols to enhance healing. The third level deals with developing spiritual consciousness and the ability to train and initiate other practitioners. All systems of Reiki share a hierarchical progression of ranks (the same as in martial arts systems): First Degree, Second Degree, and Master. The Masters are the ones who initiate the newer students as they progress upward in rank.

As with the whole array of laying-on-of-hands systems, Reiki is used to promote natural self-healing by recharging and rebalancing energy fields. A Reiki practitioner administers this energy in a meditative state with gentle laying on of hands, sometimes only hovering over the body, in a nondirected and nondiagnostic manner. A person receiving the Reiki healing method remains fully clothed and may recline, sit, or stand.

Reiki practitioners believe that Reiki improves physical and spiritual well-being, and works by influencing the neurological-endocrine-immune systems. Reiki has been used on a variety of conditions, such as strokes, seizures, fibromyalgia, childbirth, surgery, heart disease, and memory and behavioral problems.

> **Deeper connections**
>
> Many ancient systems practiced a laying on of hands for purposes other than healing. In Huna, the ancient healing and spiritual discipline of the shamans of ancient Hawaii, each master passed his gift and authority along to the next generation by the physical gesture of laying on of hands, along with a meditative transfer of energy to the initiate. Is this virtually universal action an actual transmission of energy, or is it a ritual drama to deepen the moment? Perhaps both.

Because it's so difficult to quantify the results of energy healing, it's admirable when a particular modality opens itself up to scientific scrutiny, and to its credit, Reiki is doing just that. Scientists analyzed existing scientific studies for randomization, blindness, and accountability, in order to draw definitive conclusions for support of the efficacy of Reiki. The difficulty in studying any system of energy healing is to obtain measurable results that show that the healing claims are accountable to more than just a strong belief system.

In one study, researchers reviewed almost 500 articles, and identified 12 clinical studies to investigate. Even though the studies suggested an increase in relaxation and comfort level, as well as a reduction in depression and anxiety, the researchers recommended further studies of higher quality research. This, of course, is the same as with studying anything, whether it's a new drug or an ancient healing modality.

A 2009 study found that the level of training and length of experience affected Reiki effectiveness. That is, healing energy flowing from a Reiki Master (the third level) differed significantly from that generated by a nonmaster (level one or two).

Abandoning Misconceptions

Misc.

William Teller, PhD, Stanford Professor Emeritus, wrote that it is a common misconception that the only way to fulfill the requirements of the scientific method is to be coldly and distantly objective during an experiment. Rather, it really only requires a complete description of the conditions of the protocol for anyone to reproduce the results. That means that one could set a mental or emotional bias as part of the protocol, whether positive, negative, or neutral. The key would be how this sort of thing can be measured.

It has been stated that once a Reiki practitioner has been initiated, and she has placed her hands on or near the patient, she does not have to pay attention to the healing at all. She could listen to music or read a book, for example. This idea isn't universally accepted among Reiki Masters.

One Reiki Master said she prefers to keep her mind clear and focused on the healing because she will often receive images or hunches during that session that point to areas where problems might be hidden. She also prefers not to take a history so she's open to whatever comes to her consciousness during the session.

In one example, she sensed a blockage in the intestinal area that she later learned was related to the Crohn's disease (an inflammatory bowel disease) of the patient. It isn't uncommon for a Reiki Master on her level to deal with emotional issues that are often the cause of physical problems. In our vocabulary, the more upgraded the healer's energy matrix, the higher the frequencies of energy the healer can download from the patient's energy matrix.

Therapeutic Touch

One last system of energy healing is noteworthy because it was developed by a PhD at New York University School of Nursing and has been taught to thousands of health professionals.

Therapeutic Touch, a helping technique developed by Dora Kunz, a clairvoyant, and Dr. Dolores Krieger, PhD, RN, is a means of using one's hands to focus healing energies toward an individual in need. The idea was described by Dr. Krieger as "unlocking one's natural potential to care for another human being." What a beautiful idea. Kunz believed that people could be taught how to heal. Dr. Krieger, a student of Kunz's, was able to learn to center, align with the universal healing energy of the WEB, and, with compassionate intent, project the healing energy flow to another person. The touch is an intervention, not a cure, and can be used with anyone from a premature baby to someone who is dying.

Kunz and Krieger had both worked with a powerful healer, Oscar Estabany, who was known for charging water and cotton to give to people in need of healing. Estabany believed his healing skill was a gift and couldn't really be taught. Kunz and Krieger disagreed.

A Gifted Healer

MISC.

Oscar Estabany, a Hungarian immigrant, worked with Bernard Grad, PhD, a cancer researcher at McGill University in Montreal. Through the 1960s, Grad involved Estabany in many experiments involving plants and animals. He would treat water with his hands and use it to grow plants, reduce tumors, slow their growth, etc. We'll meet him again in Chapter 10.

In the early 1970s, Therapeutic Touch was born at the Pumpkin Hollow Farm, now called the Pumpkin Hollow Retreat Center. Many of the early students were nurses, and now Therapeutic Touch has been taught to hundreds of thousands of health professionals and lay people throughout the United States, Canada, and around the world. Therapeutic Touch is accepted in a growing number of hospitals and is taught in universities at graduate levels.

Thanks to Dr. Krieger's science and medical background, research was encouraged. In her first study, Krieger found that the hemoglobin content in a person's red blood cells changed significantly after receiving a healing treatment by a Therapeutic Touch practitioner.

Research supports that Therapeutic Touch has been used successfully for a multitude of conditions. It elicits a rapid relaxation response, reduces the perception of pain, and enhances one's sense of comfort and well-being, facilitates the healing process (e.g., callus formation in bones and wounds), has a positive effect on the immune system, helps alleviate stress and anxiety, and promotes comfort in the dying process.

There are thousands of case studies that support the effectiveness of Therapeutic Touch as a complement in treating individuals with arthritis, fibromyalgia, MS, headaches, high blood pressure, side effects of chemotherapy, and diseases of the immune system.

The training system, both an art and a science, seems very methodical and will sound familiar based on what we've already covered. Students are first given activities to help them recognize that a field of energy extends beyond the skin's boundary—in our vocabulary, an energy matrix. Then they're taught to center themselves. They learn exercises designed to increase their sensitivity to energy fields, enabling a student to perform an assessment of another's energy matrix. Once energy blockages are identified, the healer proceeds to clear the congested energy and initiate the healing process.

As with all systems of energy healing, illness is seen as an imbalance in an individual's energy field, so the intention when performing Therapeutic Touch is to direct and modulate energy to re-establish a harmonious rhythmic flow and rebalance the person's energy matrix.

One of the most admirable features of Therapeutic Touch is that it has struck a balance between a traditional energy healing paradigm and a more conventional Western model involving research and testing. Moreover, with all the new technologies being introduced daily, Western medicine has gotten away from the human element of touching and caring that Therapeutic Touch attempts to restore. Balance is the key, and this gentle system does just that.

Essential Takeaways

- The most ancient form of energy healing was the laying on of hands. Virtually every ancient school of inner development had some version of this art.
- There are hundreds of variations in Qi Gung, a meditation exercise designed to evoke self-healing.
- Many of the modern systems (such as Silva, Reiki, and Therapeutic Touch) are attempting to engage the scientific research community to study their results.

chapter 8

Manual Therapy

Whole-body energy massage

Light-touch manual therapy

Energy massage through holographic access systems

Case studies in energy healing massage systems

A large number of energy healing modalities use manual therapy, ranging from light touch to deep tissue massage, as the primary means of treatment. Whether it's performed by the healer or by the patient himself, manual healing is a way of affecting the energy matrix through the soft tissue of the body. The energy blockages are embedded, so to speak, in the body, and manual modalities with an energy component provide a great way to release them.

Shiatsu

Coined at the beginning of the twentieth century in Japan, the word shiatsu means finger pressure. This system uses pressure massage from the fingers, thumbs, and palms, but also incorporates stretching exercises and some other massage techniques, depending on the school.

As with many energy healing systems, Shiatsu is based on centuries-old modalities that have been brought into modern times. Some versions of Shiatsu are more traditional, incorporating many of the tools used in TCM (Traditional Chinese Medicine) such as pulses and meridians, while other schools have attempted to incorporate Western anatomy and physiology into the practitioner's database.

Shiatsu can vary quite a bit depending on the version practiced. If you have a preference for a more modern or traditional approach, be sure to ask the right questions when you first interview your practitioner. That way you can determine if their method is the right fit for you.

Shiatsu is usually performed while the patient is clothed and on a table or futon. More traditionally used for stress reduction, relieving muscle tension and basic emotional patterns of anxiety or depression, the purpose of the massage is to locate energy blockages and reestablish the flow of ki (chi). When done properly, Shiatsu can relieve all sorts of ailments and stimulate the body's ability to heal itself.

In the more traditional schools the diagnosis precedes the massage or treatment. Chinese pulses, facial, odor, and tongue diagnosis are all utilized, along with the history-taking, to determine where the energy excesses or deficiencies lie, and then the practitioner proceeds to reestablish balance within the energy matrix. There is a concept of "diagnosis and treatment together" in Shiatsu, which seems to be a way of describing how the practitioner downloads information from the patient's energy matrix, utilizing his or her energy to facilitate the healing process. For example, if the practitioner feels a certain tension or blockage during the massage, he'll work that area or point until the body "tells" him or her that the energy is now flowing.

Acupressure and Acupuncture

Acupressure is a very powerful method for treating pressure points on your body. The only difference between acupressure and *acupuncture* is that acupressure massages the points, whereas acupuncture uses needles. Although you probably don't think of acupuncture as a system of manual therapy, it's relevant to the discussion.

The Latin word acu means needle; **acupuncture** means needle-puncture. People often think it's related to the word accurate because of the common mispronunciation, and because the placing of needles is a very accurate art. Actually, the word should be pronounced *ah-koo-puncture*, not *ah-kyoo-puncture*.

Acupuncture is the very well-known system in t'ai chi healing in which needles are inserted to points all over the body to balance the energy flow within the meridians. This serves to increase energy in places where it's deficient and to diminish energy where there's too much, often caused by energy blocks. Once the diagnostician has determined where the source of the problem lies, it's easier to select the correct points for needling (or in acupressure, massaging). Activating those needles is like opening and closing valves in a complex plumbing system to increase or decrease the flow of water.

The Chinese name for acupuncture is zhen jui, which means needle heat. This is based on the fact that needles and heat are two of the common ways to stimulate acupuncture points. But they aren't the only methods; massage is only one of the most prevalent. Different practitioners utilize other tools such as electricity, lasers, color, and even mental direction of Qi.

There's an old story that sheds some light on the similarities between acupuncture and acupressure. In ancient times, the master would look at the body and see (clairvoyantly) or feel (clairsentiently) which points needed to be palpated and mentally direct Qi to that point. The students, not being Qi Gung masters, would ask for methods that were more on their level. The master would teach them how to stimulate the point by holding a burning stick of moxa—the Chinese herb mugwort—near it. This was called Moxibustion and is still very much in use today. The students would say that Moxibustion was too difficult. "If that's still too complicated for you," the teacher said, "try palpating the point." But the students still thought it was too hard. "Okay, fine," as the acupuncture joke goes, "just stick a needle in it!"

Herbs Over Needles

Most people don't realize that in traditional Chinese medicine, acupuncture is used less often in treatment than herbal supplements; some say there's about a 70–30 percent split. Because needles are more exotic and less common in the West, they get all the press!

Whether you use heat, cold, colored light, or electro-stimulation, once you know which points to stimulate, treatment can proceed. Modern medical electro-acupuncture technology has found objective validation of acupuncture points measured in specific ranges of millivolts and micro-amps. When the meridians have an imbalance of energy, it's detected as changes in those electrical ranges.

Is there an advantage to acupressure over acupuncture? Not really, as both have advantages and disadvantages. Acupuncture is done by a professional and so may be more costly. You can do acupressure on yourself. On the other hand, the pressure may be more painful than the needles.

> **Deeper Connections**
>
> One ancient method of identifying and treating acupressure points, strangely enough, involved a quartz crystal suspended loosely inside the rib cage of a cat's skeleton. As the healer moved the devise over the body, the crystal would periodically begin to vibrate, indicating an imbalance at that location. The healer would direct his or her Qi through the crystal to amplify the energy, like shining sunlight through a magnifying glass. That was dowsing (see Chapter 9), acupuncture, and Qi Gung all at the same time.

If you plan on attempting acupressure on yourself, a professional diagnosis is the most intelligent way to begin. You wouldn't go through a drug store and randomly choose over-the-counter medications and mix them arbitrarily, and randomly choosing pressure points to massage for specific ailments is a similar idea. In Chapter 16, I explain a self-contained massage routine that balances the whole matrix without singling out any one organ or meridian. If you follow those guidelines as indicated, you can initiate a gradual balancing of your whole energy matrix. It's a good place to start.

Many self-help acupressure systems have evolved over the years, including Dr. Dale's 18-point system to balance the whole body. G-Jo was another system that was quite popular for a while. If you choose any of the books that recommend specific points as opposed to areas, be gentle in your massage at first. A single point or two may put too much emphasis on a particular channel of energy that could temporarily throw the system further out of balance.

Choosing between a system that sees the whole body as one energy matrix and one that is just a collection of points is indicative of a much bigger divide. Many medical acupuncturists who haven't had traditional acupuncture training treat points based on complex "cookbooks" that have lists of symptoms and points to needle: you look up the symptom, see what points are recommended, and needle them. More traditional acupuncturists go through deep diagnostic protocols, as discussed in Chapter 6, before they select their points. That's a much more holistic and effective approach to the healing of the energy matrix.

If you think about the word acupressure etymologically, you'll probably realize how little sense it makes. We use the term to differentiate between the use of massage and needles, but the prefix acu means needle! I like to think of the term acupressure as hyphenated, where the translation is needle-pressure, one or the other.

If you're sensitive to pain, you'll find that massage is much more uncomfortable than needles. Most of the time when the very thin acupuncture needle is inserted, you won't even feel it. Remember, the acupuncture needle is not a hollow hypodermic needle used to deliver a vaccine or Novocain or when your doctor draws blood; it's a solid piece of metal and therefore much thinner than the needles you're likely used to. A big, blunt thumb will evoke a stronger, more painful reaction.

Once inserted, the acupuncturist will gently twirl the needle back and forth between his fingers until the patient feels a slight electric shock indicating that the needle has made contact with the meridian. This is called the teh chi, which literally means obtaining the energy. The first time you experience this, it will feel a little strange. You'll look down and see the top of a needle sticking out, but you won't feel it; the rest of the needle, sometimes one or two inches' worth, are already inside you. Suddenly, with the teh chi twirl, you feel a little surge of electricity. That tells you the healer, through his manipulation of the needle, has initiated the healing process.

Once teh chi has been established and the needle has been activated, it may surprise you to know that it's very difficult to pull the needle out. Only a second before it would have slid right out and now it won't. After a few minutes, when it's done its balancing work, the needle can be removed without any resistance at all. It seems to know when its job is done and it's ready to come out. It sounds amazing, but that's how it works!

The choice of needles or pressure is up to you. Either way, learning to massage the areas that balance the whole body's energy matrix (that I mentioned previously) is always a good idea. I developed one such chart and call it the RB (Reflex Balance) everyday areas and you'll learn how to do that self-massage in Chapter 16.

Craniosacral Therapy

Craniosacral therapy (CST) is a system that seeks to reestablish the flow and pressure of the cerebrospinal fluid in and around the head and spine, cranium referring to the head, sacrum to the base of the spine. Because the brain and spinal cord form the structure of the central nervous system (and some of the very important control organs within the brain, such as the pituitary and pineal glands and the hypothalamus), changes in the rhythm of that fluid can have serious consequences.

In anatomical terms, the craniosacral system is composed of the support structure of the bones of the spine and skull, the brain and spinal cord within, the cerebrospinal fluid that bathes it, and the membranes (meninges) that surround it. Just as we have a pulse and heartbeat, we also have a craniosacral rhythm. According to many holistic practitioners, this rhythm is generated by pressure changes caused by the ebb and flow of the cerebrospinal fluid.

The premise in craniosacral therapy is that an infant's experience of birth, head injury, problems in other parts of the body, or trauma during life can throw this system out of balance, and impede the proper rhythm and flow needed for the body to heal itself.

The craniosacral therapist uses very gentle palpation of the skull, sacrum, and spine to sense the motion and pulse of this rhythm, isolate points of restriction, and correct them.

Osteopathic physicians have been doing this sort of manipulation for quite some time, focusing more on the manipulation of the cranial bones or plates. John Upledger, DO, OMM, founded craniosacral therapy, focusing more on the manipulation of the underlying meninges or membranes, which frees the restrictions found in the cranium, ribs, and spinal column.

Finding Meaning

Osteopaths use the knowledge of the structure (anatomy) and function (physiology) of the body and apply it to all diseases, disorders, and dysfunctions. Through a comprehensive evaluation of a person's biomechanics, the osteopath can determine where the imbalances lie and restore its function using a variety of safe, gentle manual techniques.

Because there's still great movement and flexibility within the cranial plates at a young age, this therapy is very effective on infants and children. Also, the results of a difficult birth are not set and locked within the system yet. There are many reported improvements in ear infections and other childhood ailments with this therapy.

A further development by Dr. Upledger and his team led to Somato-Emotional Release, an even subtler therapy that releases underlying emotional trauma. Injuries and shocks to the system lead to the formation of "energy cysts" that prevent the body from functioning at full efficiency. Referring back to our common vocabulary, energy cysts are the energy blocks that manifest on the psycho-emotional frequency of our energy matrix. This therapy works to free those blockages.

When you watch a CST therapist at work, it appears to be almost a laying on of hands at times. The touch of the therapist is extremely gentle, almost hovering over the areas. Clearly, the therapist has phase-locked with the patient and learned to listen with her fingers to these most subtle rhythms.

Remember that in the Chinese pulse system, there are many types of questions you can ask the body to get information. Here, too, the craniosacral rhythm has a wealth of information if you know how to download it.

A parallel system of spinal massage is found in t'ai chi healing and is thousands of years old. The YU system, a series of points along the spine and skull (along the urinary bladder meridian), is utilized for treating the whole body. All meridians and organs in the body are linked to the YU system and, by manipulation of these points, the entire body can be treated. While there is no direct relationship between the YU system and CST, both utilize the spine to access the whole energy matrix.

Zone Therapy and Reflexology

As you learned in Chapter 6, there are two major types of acupuncture/acupressure systems, labeled by Dr. Dale as macro-acupuncture and micro-acupuncture—the latter of which we called the holographic access systems. To refresh your memory, the macro systems, used in traditional acupuncture and Shiatsu, incorporate the 14 major meridians that traverse the entire body. The holographic access systems, on the other hand, are found on a particular finite anatomical location: ears, eyes, hands, feet, etc.

Each of these holographic access systems, the most famous being the feet, can access the entire database of the energy matrix.

The modern system of massage that became Zone Therapy and foot reflexology began in the early twentieth century with William Fitzgerald, MD, and his followers. He discovered a relationship between longitudinal zones in the body and related reflex zones in the hands, feet, face, etc., and developed a system based on the following premises:

Within the electromagnetic fields of the body, there are both longitudinal and latitudinal force lines that can be used to create a grid. The first thing to do is to firmly establish the location of that grid and to plot the various organs on it.

If you take a single holographic unit, such as the two feet held together, and place the electromagnetic grid over it, you can map the organs and body parts onto the grid and even draw a small human modified somewhat to fit into the different-shaped contour of the feet.

The theory is that by stimulating a particular reflex point on the feet, you can affect the related organ or anatomical body part.

Fitzgerald found he could stimulate these corresponding reflexes with pressure to produce analgesia and therapeutic effects. He called this early system Zone Therapy.

Over the next few decades, his followers and their students began to experiment with these maps and were able to produce all sorts of therapeutic results. Eunice Ingham, a student and colleague of Dr. Fitzgerald, coined the term reflexology in the 1930s. Mildred Carter popularized reflexology with her best-selling book, *Helping Yourself with Foot Reflexology*.

Not every chart maps the organs in the same way. Some charts will even place the same organ on completely different sides of the various holographic access systems. As different practitioners experienced different results, they often mapped the holographic access systems differently.

This is generally not viewed as problematic; if the healer's intention is to send energy to a particular organ, the energy goes to that organ, whether the right reflex connection was palpated or not. Besides, reflexologists generally massage the entire foot as part of the session, so all the reflexes are stimulated, even with opposing maps.

Every System Evolves

Misc.

Science and energy healing are in a constant state of evolution. We are always discovering new information about how the body works and why some therapies work. Don't look at older charts as being inaccurate; rather, they are simply indicative of a perfectly valid phase of the evolution of the practice.

The following charts show a more contemporary model of anatomical organs overlaid on the holographic access system of the hands and feet known as RB (Reflex Balance).

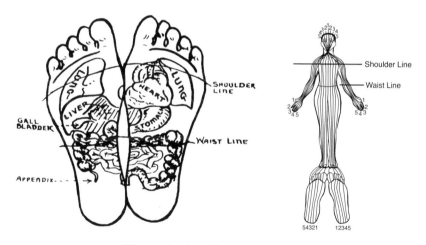

Fitzgerald's original Zone Therapy grids.

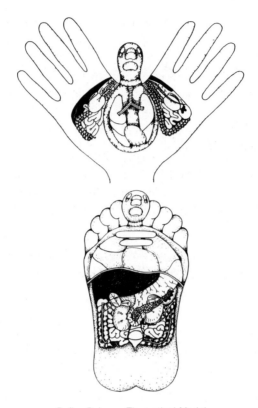

Reflex Balance-Theoretical Model.

Case Studies in Energy Healing Through Massage

In many healing cases, it takes time to uncover the cause, whether physical, emotional, or spiritual. If you can figure out the exact nature of the energy block, the problem can be solved more quickly. Here are a few cases where the referred pain or symptom was linked to an old energy block, and through manual therapy, a quick positive result occurred. Almost any of the systems we've discussed in this chapter could achieve these types of results in the right hands.

The Retired Dancer

A retired professional ballet dancer was suffering with severe leg pain in the gluteus maximus muscles. She'd had minimal discomfort during her years dancing in New York but figured the pain would go away once she retired. Not only had it not gone away, it had become much worse. She explained that she now taught classes in her own school and was becoming more and more incapacitated by the pain.

Considering the demands that professional dance has on the body, it was no surprise that she had the pain to begin with. She was hoping to alleviate some of that pain, assuming she hadn't done permanent damage to the joint.

When she arrived, she was wearing a leotard that revealed the upper end of a scar that began at her chest bone. She explained that she'd had cosmetic surgery to her chest bone; she was born with an indented chest cavity and, for the purpose of professional ballet cosmetics, she'd had it corrected early in her career. When asked whether the leg pain dated to the time of her chest surgery, she realized they had indeed happened at the same time. The connection had never occurred to her before.

The key connection: The gluteus maximus muscles, where the pain was felt, are related to the *pericardium* meridian.

Finding Meaning

The **pericardium** is the physical double-walled sac around the heart. It's one of the primary meridians in t'ai chi healing and is associated with the circulation of sexual energy. It's also paired with the triple-warmer meridian that's related to the endocrine glands or, according to other theories, to the respiratory, digestive, and excretory organs.

After a few moments of palpation, she got up and moved around. The pain, which had plagued her for years, was gone. The connection: surgery to the chest had affected the physical pericardium; the physical pericardium trickled up and caused an energy imbalance in the pericardium meridian; the energy imbalance caused a message to be sent, via the meridian, to the gluteus muscles in the leg. The chest had healed years ago, but the energy scar in the pericardium had remained. The healing broke up the energy block through the palpation of the appropriate reflex point; the pain disappeared and didn't return.

The Corporate Executive

The CEO of a large corporation hired me to do a stress management course for their upper-level executives. (This is somewhat ironic, considering the upper-level execs are usually the ones *causing* the stress for the middle management, who probably need the training more.) The CEO listened politely (and somewhat skeptically) and asked whether this sort of thing could help his right arm, which he had been unable to lift past the horizontal level since suffering a bike accident 16 years earlier.

The spinal source in the neck for all the nerves that go down the arms is called the brachial plexus in basic anatomy, which is linked in energy healing to the fifth chakra. After 20 seconds of palpation to the RB points related to the fifth chakra on each of his hands, he was able to lift his arm straight up to 12 o'clock, with no pain at all! The problem never returned.

The Boy with Tinnitus

A 10-year-old boy was suffering with tinnitus, or ringing in his ears. Doctors had been unable to eliminate it. One physician suggested that the cause might be psychological. A healer, though, looks for other, less-obvious causes. Turns out, this boy had undergone surgery for an undescended testicle at birth. That's a pretty common and simple procedure, but the surgery could have impacted the urinary bladder meridian, which, in acupuncture's five-element theory, is related to the ear. It was a long shot, but the healer massaged the urinary bladder meridian on the foot and the ringing stopped.

The Skeptical MD

At the suggestion of a colleague, a highly skeptical professor of pediatrics sought energy healing for upper back and shoulder pain. In cases like this, the holographic access system of the feet would normally show tremendous tension in the back and shoulder areas, but in this case, the reflexes to her spine and shoulders were so flexible and loose that they almost seemed too relaxed. That blew the MD patient away, because she hadn't yet stated the cause of her pain. As it turned out she had a congenital disease in which her bones were "soft" and had even had a metal rod implanted surgically to keep her spine from collapsing.

In addition to that problem, there was a tremendous energy imbalance in her kidneys. When the healer asked the patient if she had any kidney problems, her colleague chimed in that there was nothing wrong with her friend's kidneys. The patient, however, interrupted her to reveal that she, in fact, had serious kidney problems and was on medication for them and had never bothered to mention it to her since the medication kept the problem under control. Nevertheless, it still manifested as an imbalance on the energy level. That incident changed the doctor from a skeptic to a lifelong student of yoga and healing.

The Neonatal Infant

In Chapter 5, I addressed the question of whether you have to believe in energy healing for it to work. This final case study involved a 36-week premature infant who clearly didn't operate from any belief system. The infant was born by emergency C-section with a good Apgar score and was sent to the normal newborn nursery. After about an hour, she developed tachypnea, with a respiratory rate up to 150 breaths per minute (bpm) and a high heart rate of 250.

The next day, while the conversion from fetal type circulation to adult pulmonary circulation was taking place, the pediatrician (an energy healer in training) thought of using RB (Reflex Balance) in an attempt to accelerate the stabilization of pulmonary circulation and lower the respiratory rate. She applied RB to the heart-lung reflexes of the infant within the incubator using soft touch pressure, as that was as much as the baby could tolerate.

stay Grounded

If you become a healer, be careful when working on acute cases where conventional medical intervention may be required. Specialized training for that is available in many healing systems, but be sure to work within the boundaries of what you've been trained for.

After 60–90 seconds of gentle RB applied to the feet of the infant, the respiratory rate dropped to 60–80 bpm. After 2 minutes of RB, the respirations dropped to as much as 40 bpm. Within 30 seconds after stopping RB, it rose to 80–90 bpm. The respiratory rate rose to a maximum 150 bpm between massages.

This was repeated on each of five RB applications at the start of every half hour, each resulting in the same changes. Nonrelated reflex points were attempted as a control but did not get the results the correct RB points did. On the sixth attempt, the breathing rate came down as it had before but respirations stayed below 110 bpm even between RB massages. After two or three more applications of RB, the baby was put on room air; soon after, the catheters were removed and the patient was transferred to the normal nursery for routine care.

Essential Takeaways

- Manual therapy systems are among the most easily accessible modalities of energy healing.
- Unlike modern-day massage, massage systems in energy healing are directed at balancing the energy matrix and not just relaxing the muscles.
- Some energy manual modalities are applied to the whole body while others only palpate or massage a specific holographic access system, such as the feet or hands.
- Some manual techniques are painful, while others are not. Choose whatever you're comfortable with.
- Manual therapies can often be used to treat symptoms that are referred from elsewhere in the body or the energy matrix.

chapter 9

Healers with Tools

Ancient and modern tools used by energy healers

Musical vibrations for energy healing

Hypnosis: energy healing through words

In addition to the many systems we've discussed that use the hands, there are a number of systems in which the healer uses some device or tool for energy diagnosis and treatment. These tools might include crystals, precious stones, pendulums, or dowsing rods. Today, technological advances have added even more to the mix, such as electro-acupuncture machines and radionics boxes. Let's take a look inside that energy healing tool kit.

Two Categories of Tools

There are two primary categories of tools that healers might use: the first are those that have some natural healing or energy property built into them and the second are those that the healer programs after she has them in her possession.

The first category is easy to understand. An herb growing naturally will have a unique energy signature and may be useful for a specific kind of problem. T'ai chi healing has an unending array of such natural remedies, as do indigenous healing systems in every culture in the world.

The second may be a little more difficult to understand. These are objects that healers treat as storage devices for their thoughts and intentions, uploading information to them as we would to a computer microchip. Often, the object has certain natural healing properties making it more receptive to the healer's energy, but unlike the herb, they need the healer's input to work.

Furthermore, some objects in the latter category are more receptive to certain types of energy than others. A simple quartz crystal found in nature may have some natural healing property within it, but it may have a different vibratory tendency than an amethyst or a rose or jade crystal. In those cases, the healer may add a certain programming to the crystal to personalize it for a particular patient or to use it either diagnostically or in treatment.

Deeper
Connections

Everything in nature has its own energy signature. Amethysts are known for their soothing and calming influence and are used for gout, insomnia, and developing mental clarity and clairvoyance. When they are warmed, wrapped in silk, and bound about the temples, they reduce headache throbbing and relieve pain and tension. Amethyst also makes someone gentler and heals with tenderness. According to ancient Egyptian belief, amethyst rays even warded off the evil eye!

The key thing to remember is that all healing energy is downloaded from the WEB, whether it's embedded in an object naturally or whether we program it in. The ability to direct one's energy intention to the patient or direct it to a tool to help the patient is an important skill for an energy healer.

Why Use Tools?

There are a number of reasons why a healer would choose to use tools rather than sending energy to a patient directly. Our minds aren't like lasers; we can't always turn them on, aim them, and produce focused energy, unaffected by distractions in the environment. Thoughts arise, phones ring in the distance; many things can distract a healer. If you're utilizing a physical object, it can help keep the mind on the task at hand. Bona fide psychics who use crystal balls don't believe the answers they seek are in the crystal; the answers are within their mind. The crystal just helps to quiet and aim the mind.

Showing the patient how to palpate a specific massage point will often get a better result than just telling him to think lovely thoughts about his life. By giving a patient a crystal to meditate on or a tea leaf to brew, you can empower him to take an active role in his own healing. Something tangible can often help in the healing.

Another example where tools can be quite effective is when the patient lives far away and can only see the healer intermittently. The healer can give the patient an object that can help him feel a little closer, as if there's a link between them. This isn't just a token. A bottle of charged water, for example, can help a patient continue the flow of energy from the healing work even when he's gone home.

Crystals and Stones

There are volumes of ancient lore about crystals and gemstones and their capacity to do everything from healing hemorrhoids to guaranteeing victory in battle to making someone fall in love.

While some of the claims may seem outlandish at first, if you look at the evolution of modern science, the effectiveness of crystals seems much more reasonable. We've learned that massive amounts of information can be stored on microscopic silicon chips. Video and audiotape, flash drives, and nanotechnology are all able to store electromagnetic signals and information. We've also seen the effects that thoughts and words can have on water, as documented by Dr. Emoto's water crystals, supporting the idea that physical objects found in nature are able to store information transmitted from our healing energy matrix. It's strange to think about, but if looked at from that perspective, there's only a very fine line between healing crystals and nanotechnology.

MISC.

Crystal Processors

All the information stored on tiny microscopic chips are just our primitive way of simulating what the brain does as it stores and transmits information. Our technology today, as advanced as it is, is like cave painting when compared to the advanced word-processors of our minds. Technology is striving to catch up and understand what we've been doing all along. Energy healers, meanwhile, may use crystals to accomplish some of these uploading and downloading tasks.

There was a case where a lively woman in her mid-50s was having symptoms of disorientation and low energy. These symptoms were very surprising because, as both she and her husband attested, she had always been a very active, high-energy type. When I was preparing to take her Chinese pulses and begin palpation on her hands, I asked her to take off her rings. She wore two huge gemstones, one on each hand that I admired as she put them aside. As I proceeded through the healing, I noticed that her energy seemed backward in a way. It's difficult to explain, but it felt as if where energy should be coming into the body, it was going out and vice versa. It was sort of like having the faucets for hot and cold water switched, the hot faucet putting out cold water and the cold putting out hot. The energy seemed confused.

I proceeded to balance her energy matrix as best I could and gave her some self-massage and breathing homework. After the balancing we chatted for a while, and then she reached for the rings to put them back on. As she took the rings, I asked if I could see them for a moment. Like all natural gemstones, these large, jeweled crystals had very distinct energies: one felt very yang (forceful, outgoing, pushing) and the other felt very yin (forcefully pulling in energy like a black hole, incoming, sucking). One pulled my scanning hand inward toward the crystal; the other pushed it away. One was like a vacuum cleaner and one was like a fire hose. Though the specific properties of these types of gemstones aren't necessarily repellant, these particular stones' individual energies were polar opposites.

Traditionally, energy enters the energy matrix on the left side of the body and is transmitted outwardly on the right. It turned out she was wearing the outgoing stone on the incoming hand and the incoming stone on the outgoing hand. The influence of these huge crystals that she wore all the time was, in effect, jamming her energy flow and causing her disorientation and low energy.

A few days after switching the rings, she couldn't believe the difference. She woke up with more energy than she'd had in a year. She also realized that the symptoms began just after her birthday, when her husband had given her the second ring.

Feeling Crystal Energy

The next time you're at a store that sells quartz crystals, empty your mind, ground yourself (see Chapter 14), and energize your hands. Then pick up one crystal at a time and scan it, as explained in Chapter 17. You'll be amazed at the sensations you feel between the crystals. If one really "talks" to you, buy it. Take it home, put it in the sun all day to cleanse it, and take it out each day to practice feeling its energy.

There are many healers who are very accomplished with crystals. They aim their thoughts through the crystals and do some amazing work, breaking up energy blocks and soothing energy scars. But remember, the tool doesn't do all the work by itself. Crystals are a powerful tool only in the hands of a well-trained healer.

Dowsing

Dowsing rods bring to mind scraggly-bearded prospectors looking for gold or oil in the Old West. The basic idea of dowsing is to hold a free-floating object (a dowsing rod, a pendulum, etc.), ask a yes-or-no question, and keep your mind open to receive the answer from the way the object moves in your hand. Similar to crystals, there's nothing in the dowsing rod or pendulum that's inherently special; it's the consciousness of the practitioner that makes the device come alive.

The art of dowsing has tremendous healing applications, which we'll explore further in Chapter 17.

A healer I knew used a loose-hanging amethyst pendulum to assess the chakras. She held it over each one and gauged whether the chakras were too yin or too yang by the way the crystal rotated, clockwise or counter-clockwise. Then she would send a healing intent through the crystal to balance the problem. The crystal hung in perfect stillness for a moment and then began to rotate. The movement indicated that the chakra was balanced and it was time to move on to the next one.

Because dowsing is about asking yes-or-no questions and then quieting yourself enough to hear the answer, the applications of the art are limitless—you just have to know what question to ask!

One evening in the late 1970s, Christopher Bird, co-author of *The Secret Life of Plants* and author of *The Divining Hand: The 500-Year-Old Mystery of Dowsing* was at a dinner party. Another guest hadn't yet arrived, and in the days before cell phones there was no way to reach him to make sure he hadn't encountered problems on a cold, rainy night.

Not having a pendulum or other dowsing implement handy, Chris brought his forefinger to the top of his other hand and began to slowly rub it back and forth. After a moment he said, "Don't worry. He's fine. He'll be here in about 12 minutes." And sure enough, exactly 12 minutes later, the other guest arrived at the house.

Chris explained that he'd programmed the sliding of his finger as a yes/no answering device. If the finger slid smoothly over his hand, the answer was no. As soon as his finger started to stick rather than slide smoothly, it was yes. He began to ask himself a series of questions. "Will he be here in 1 minute? Will he be here in 2 minutes?" As he counted higher and higher, he kept getting negative answers until he got to 12. Then his finger stuck to his hand. "He'll be here in 12 minutes."

The obvious question is whether he really needed the finger to ask and answer the question. Wasn't it just a psychic phenomenon like telepathy or clairvoyance? The answer was that, yes, he could have asked the question without it, but he felt the use of dowsing, after many years, helped clear and focus his mind. That's the key to dowsing, and to energy healing: keeping the mind clear and focused so you can be receptive to the energy.

Electro-Acupuncture Machines

When teaching acupuncture, Dr. Ralph Alan Dale encouraged the use of electro-acupuncture machines. He felt that once you accessed the teh chi, the use of a device that could put a continuous stream of electricity through the needle would stimulate the point more evenly. You would simply attach a small alligator clip to the end of the needle, set the specific frequency and rhythm of the current, and let 'er rip! These devices definitely stimulate the points! Sometimes the needle even dances around a bit because of the electricity going through it.

stay Grounded

Energy healing machines are an area of study unto themselves. You need to learn all the settings of the dials that put out different energy distribution patterns, as well as increments of current. It's a very specific science. If it interests you, be sure to learn it from a qualified expert and not someone who dabbles with acupuncture "toys" or learned it from a manual.

You might think that using machines takes the healer out of the healing process. While this is a legitimate concern, you can't just put the needles in, hook them up to the machine, and forget about the contact between you and the patient. Here is a very sad case that illustrates just how necessary the healer's involvement is, even when working with machines.

The patient was a man who had gone up to the roof to fetch his 5-year-old son's balloon from a tree branch. Holding on to the TV antenna, he reached out as far as he could with a golf-ball retriever, but at that very moment there was some switch in polarity, as he described it, in the nearby electrical cable that caused a giant surge of electricity that arced between the power line and the antenna. He was in the middle of it, ungrounded, and literally lit up like a light bulb. His arms were scorched beyond repair and both had to be amputated at the elbows.

Over a year later, the problem was his phantom limb pain. It wasn't just the pain at the point of amputation, where some of the nerves had grown and were firing as they contacted each other like open electrical wires. He actually felt pain where his fingers and the parts of his arm that had been amputated had been. Some folks in conventional medicine say that phantom pain is psychological. Energy healers tend to think there's a real energy component present, that the limb still exists within the energy matrix, even if it's physically gone. Either way, he was experiencing severe hand and finger pain where there were no hands.

When I sat at his feet and pressed RB points related to a specific finger, the pain in that phantom finger stopped. When the pressure was released, the pain returned. We were all quite excited and optimistic! Unfortunately, even though the palpation relieved the pain during the session, it couldn't keep the pain away. It came back soon after.

We decided to try using an electro-acupuncture machine to produce the same result as the palpation. If it worked, we planned on designing a portable *transcutaneous electrical nerve stimulation (TENS)* unit to give him relief throughout the day, matching the frequency of the device to produce anesthesia.

Finding Meaning

A **transcutaneous electrical nerve stimulation (TENS)** unit provides therapeutic electrical nerve stimulation. It can be made as a portable, battery-operated unit that puts out the same pattern of electricity as an electro-acupuncture machine.

Electro-acupuncture as an anesthetizing agent had been used in China for years when performing open-heart surgery. When testing it with this patient, however, it had absolutely no effect whatsoever. The pain could only be relieved by human palpation, and then it wouldn't last.

Dr. Puharich hypothesized that the phantom limb pain was at a much higher frequency within the energy matrix. The machine could handle the slower frequencies of meridians, which are much closer to the physical nerves in our bodies, but not the etheric energies, the word he used to describe the faster frequencies of the energy matrix.

Clearly modern technological tools are helpful, but they can't replace the energy and intent of a healer.

Radionics and the Black Box

Another healing approach that utilizes what appears to be an electronic device is radionics. The idea is that a hair or blood sample—something with the energy signature of the patient—is placed in the small cup within an electronic box. The sample in the cup creates an energy link with the patient. The healer phase-locks with the patient and turns a series of dials on the box until she feels she has reached the correct frequency for each particular chakra, much like a dowser asking a question and awaiting an answer.

Far from Far Fetched

When you hear about using a strand of hair or a blood sample, it starts sounding like turn-of-the-twentieth-century medical quackery or witchcraft. You might even be picturing Professor Snape hovering over a smoldering cauldron. But if you think about it, taking a single cell of an organism, utilizing its DNA sequencing, and cloning a copy of it, sounds more far-fetched than balancing chakras using a piece of hair.

The sample will be on the frequency of the person's energy signature; with radionics a healer can tune into it, diagnose it (or determine the status of a chakra), and then send a healing intent to the patient through the machine. Here, again, it's only a tool to get the healer to focus.

Music for Healing

While music is the least tangible of the healing tools, it is an amazingly powerful way to alter your mood, boost your energy, or put you in a particular frame of mind. To take it a step further, music is vibration, and vibration is what energy healing is all about.

You may have seen science experiments in which certain types of music are played to plants. Some plants grow toward the speakers while others grow away. Dr. Emoto has done extensive testing with music and water; you can guess how water crystals feel about Mozart versus death metal.

There was a study conducted back in the 1970s in which the wires in speakers were disconnected so there was no audible sound, though the effect of the vibrations of the music on the plants remained the same. Nature knows which vibrations are conducive to harmony and balance and which aren't.

Some musicians have learned how to tap into this reality to use music for healing. Dr. Stephen Halpern, PhD, is a master musician and composer. His music, well-known throughout the New Age world, has profound results in energy healing. Over 30 years ago, he spoke of how the 5 notes of the pentatonic scale in music, as opposed to our familiar 7-note scale, are part of the source for music healing. There's a silent sixth note that one can hear only with one's inner ear, similar to the inner third eye spoken about by mystics and meditators. If you can tap into that vibration, energy healing can naturally take place. To this day, many healers quietly play Dr. Halpern's music during healing sessions.

Hypnosis

Hypnosis is an ancient art that's a viable tool in guiding patients to greater wellness. It can be used to help patients achieve an 8 hz state that enables them to log on to the WEB. Whether you call it guided imagery, guided relaxation, imagery rehearsal, meditation, or even deep prayer, all are variations on hypnosis.

The word hypnosis, coined in 1841, is rooted in the Greek word for sleep, hypnos. This is somewhat misleading, as the trance state isn't sleep at all. In fact, most of us are in a trance state quite often—when we daydream, watch TV, or during prolonged highway driving.

In an 8 hz state, one is able to direct change within the energy matrix and thereby stimulate the body's self-healing systems. What the hypnotherapist calls establishing rapport with the subject is what we have been calling phase-locking the energy matrix of the healer with that of the patient. The words of the hypnotherapist are the energies of healing.

Perspectives on Hypnosis

There are many misconceptions about hypnosis. For years it has been abused as a stage show trick, with people afraid they'll be made to do things against their will under hypnosis. The truth is, hypnosis is merely a method of accessing a deeper level of the mind. Subjects remain in complete control of themselves at all times. No one can be hypnotized unwillingly; hypnotic suggestibility is based on the willingness and trust of the subject.

In hypnosis, the body is deeply relaxed and the brain waves are in the alpha state, which is slower than the alert state (beta) but above deep sleep (delta) or even deeper meditation (theta). Persons in hypnotic trance are fully aware of their surroundings, but their attention is deliberately focused on something in order to distract them from something else, such as pain. This has many applications in clinical practice, including dentistry, obstetrics, oncology, and trauma care.

In my first hypnosis class, I told the teacher I had never been hypnotized; my mind was probably too busy thinking about the process. After the induction and emergence from trance, when he brought everyone back to an awake state by counting one-two-three, he asked me how I'd done. I said I thought I had fallen asleep. If so, he asked, why had I opened my eyes on three? He was right; not only had I been in a deeper trance than I thought, but I was aware of everything he had said.

Hypnotherapy is not a cure-all; in fact, it isn't actually a cure at all, though it can be an effective tool for alleviating subjective symptoms. The underlying cause of the symptoms must still be identified and treated. While the effects of hypnosis are widely recognized, its mechanism is unknown. The link between a verbal suggestion and a physiological response hasn't been identified, but medical science believes it's probably via the limbic system of the brain. Many healers, myself included, feel there's an energy aspect to the process as well.

Hypnosis and Medicine

In the early 1850s, before the discovery of chloroform, hypnotic trance, called mesmerism at the time, was successfully used for surgical anesthesia. Dr. James Esdaile was the first to use hypnosis for surgery while working in India. He performed over 300 major operations and thousands of minor ones without the use of chemical anesthesia. Dr. John Elliotson also used this procedure, though both fell into disrepute because of considerable opposition.

Mesmerizing

The origins of modern hypnosis date back to the 1770s, when Dr. Franz Anton Mesmer formulated his theory of animal magnetism. Dr. Mesmer didn't call it hypnosis and never realized that his results were obtained by what we now call hypnotic suggestion. However, his legacy lives on; the word "mesmerized" comes from his early form of hypnosis.

Sigmund Freud used hypnosis in his psychoanalysis treatment, though eventually stopped, declaring that symptomatic treatment was ineffective in the long run. Milton H. Erickson, MD, is widely recognized as the foremost hypnotherapist of the last century. He was instrumental in the formal recognition of hypnosis by a number of medical associations.

The British Medical Association formally accepted hypnosis as a safe and effective modality of medical treatment in 1955. Soon after, the American Dental Association and the American Medical Association formally accepted it as well.

Besides allaying pain, hypnotherapy is now being used to treat the symptoms of asthma, arthritis, Parkinsonism, migraines, depression, phobias, addictions, bulimia, insomnia, hypertension, nausea, gastric hyperacidity, burns, and skin disorders, as well as weight loss and smoking cessation.

While under general anesthesia or in a coma, patients are cognitively receptive, and auditory input is absorbed at the subconscious level. This can be a powerful healing tool. Bart Ostroff, MA, CMH, for example, a master hypnotherapist, created audiotapes for patients to listen to via headphones during surgery. These tapes, customized to the patient and the medical procedure involved, instill suggestions that minimize pain, promote healing, and hasten recovery time.

As for the psychological realm, Ostroff once hypnotized a patient with a cat phobia so severe that she'd cross the street if she saw one coming. In trance, she discovered her fears traced back to her early childhood in Ethiopia, where witches and cats were linked. Under hypnosis, she reframed this past programming. At her next session, a month later, she informed Ostroff she had bought two kittens!

Dr. Erickson recognized that most people rely on the limited capacities of their conscious mind, even though the unconscious contains much more information and resources about the world around them. Moreover, because each person draws upon the past and creates solutions to problems differently, the approach to solving problems will be different.

Rather than have the same inductions and suggestions for each patient, which directly suggest how to re-model his thinking or re-direct his energy, Erikson's strategy was a more indirect approach. His language was nondirective in style. For instance, he'd say, "I wonder if you'll be surprised to notice …," or "If you can let yourself be aware of …."

He spoke in stories and metaphors, which would contain guidance within them. He was a genius at linking the characters in the metaphors to a patient's situation, finishing the story in such a way that the characters would resolve a conflict and achieve their desired outcome. He helped his patients find solutions to their problems by accessing resources from their own subconscious within the context of the story.

Pay the Cashier

There's a famous story about a man who came to Dr. Erikson to help him quit smoking. Erikson chatted with the man for about an hour and then told him the session was over and to pay the cashier $500 on the way out. When the man said he hadn't even been hypnotized yet, Erikson asked him if he had any desire for a cigarette. The man thought for a second and realized he didn't. Erikson smiled and said, "Pay the cashier!"

Both modern and traditional hypnosis are part of the art of captivating a patient's attention and, in doing so, therapeutically communicating ideas that motivate subjects to change their perception.

Essential Takeaways

- Healers can utilize physical tools to help them focus their minds during a healing.
- Healers can use music to access the right vibrations for energy healing.
- Hypnosis can be a powerful tool to alter how we process information and access both the subconscious and the energy matrix.

chapter 10

Energy Healing with Plants, Food, and Drink

Macrobiotics: food for energy healing

Ayurvedic and homeopathic healing

Water for energy healing

We've looked at some healing systems involving touch and seen some of the additional tools and objects healers use to help them in the healing process. There's another kind of tool that stands apart as a category unto itself, focusing on tools we ingest: the plants and herbs we take for medication, the food we eat, even the water we drink, all of which play a prominent role in the world of energy healing.

Macrobiotics

Certain diets are designed to balance the energy matrix, the most well known being macrobiotics. Modern macrobiotics, literally meaning "large life," is a dietary system developed by George Ohsawa and further refined by Michio Kushi, although there are ancient forerunners to the approach as far back as ancient Greece. The basic idea is that by eating certain foods in a certain way, you can keep the yin/yang polarity of the energy matrix in balance.

The first step is to diagnose the condition of your energy matrix and then properly select the foods that will restore balance and therefore encourage your body to heal itself.

If your body, for example, has an excess of yin energy, you could restore balance by eating the right yang foods, as all foods can be characterized as either yin or yang. This oversimplified description is a lot more complicated than it sounds. The diagnosis is based on which organs and meridians are excessive or deficient of energy. Kushi believes that even cancer is caused by an imbalance of yin and yang dietary choices.

stay Grounded

It's not uncommon for people to read a book or two on macrobiotics and believe they can diagnose themselves. In fact, if they do this improperly, they can throw their system further out of balance. In addition, transitioning to a macrobiotic diet isn't a simple affair. It should all be one handled under the guidance of an expert guide.

In addition to the diagnostic and dietary specifics, Kushi recommends specific dietary practices: chewing food thoroughly and mixing it well with saliva, eating at least three hours before going to bed, and not overeating. These, combined with the yin-yang dietary balance, help create a more peaceful and balanced energy matrix. Whether you practice macrobiotics or not, that's good advice.

Ayurvedic Medicine

The quintessential system of yoga healing is known as Ayurvedic medicine. The word Ayurvedic means "science of long life" and the system itself is thousands of years old. It is estimated that up to 80 percent of India's current population uses some traditional healing modality. Ayurvedic medicine has recently achieved popularity in the West thanks to the popular writings of Dr. Deepak Chopra.

Ayurvedic medicine isn't a system that focuses on disease but rather on the individual. Once you understand a person, you can determine the cause of disease and guide him or her to a lifestyle that will prevent future illness.

Ayurvedic medicine is a holistic system that strives for the balance of body, mind, and spirit. To achieve that harmony, it utilizes diverse strategies, including diet, yoga, breathing exercises, meditation, massage, chanting, herbal remedies, baths, tonics, inhalations, enemas, and more.

The principle underlying Ayurvedic medicine is this: Everything in the world is composed of five elements (air, fire, ether, water, and earth), similar to the five-element theory of t'ai chi healing but with slightly different elements. The never-ending interplay of these energies results in different combinations that determine the patient's metabolic type.

Each one of us has one of three major metabolic types or doshas: vata (air/ether, governing communication and movement), pitta (fire/water, governing transformation, metabolism, and digestion), and kapha (water/earth, governing stability and structure). In addition to the different body types these reflect (thin, muscular, or heavy), there are mental, emotional, and spiritual distinctions that separate the types. Each individual is a unique combination of these elements and doshas, although we are predominantly one of the three.

Although this can seem complicated to a beginner, the basic idea is that whatever type we are, when we aren't in balance, our body will be susceptible to disease. Ayurveda outlines the seven main factors that can destroy our balance: genetic, congenital, internal, seasonal, electromagnetic, external trauma, and natural habits.

The Power of Ten

Misc.

Remember the tree of life, the t'ai chi t'u, and the quarks of string theory side by side in Chapter 3? All these models suggest that, on some level of our energy matrix, we're defined by an infinite interplay of 10 component lights or particles. In each of these diagrams, we see the 10 components in 3 arrays of 3, with a tenth free-floating one that somehow links them together. Perhaps the Ayurvedic metabolic types are one more manifestation of this complex energy relationship.

The diagnosis process in Ayurvedic medicine will sound familiar: taking pulses and observing the tongue, eyes, and nails, as well as detailed urine examination. Nowadays, among some Ayurvedic practitioners, a number of technological diagnostic tools are joining the more ancient ones as well.

Once diagnosed, the patient must undergo detoxification, tonification, rejuvenation, and, finally, mental and spiritual elevation through self-discipline, all utilizing some or all of the strategies listed previously.

Ayurvedic medicine strives toward a deeper level of spiritual awareness and aims for a purer kind of living. It's an ancient system of healing and growth, encompassing the physical, mental, and spiritual dimensions of humanity. It urges each of us to become fully functional as a purified energy matrix, to learn to log on to the WEB, and to surf as high and as freely as we can.

Homeopathy: Water Plus Energy

Samuel Heinemann developed homeopathy in the late eighteenth century. The word homeopathy means "similar suffering," and a homeopathic remedy is prescribed based upon its ability to mimic the disease state, thereby stimulating the body to heal itself. Homeopathy considers the body's own defense system to be the optimal healing system. The homeopathic remedy stimulates these defenses to work more effectively.

Homeopathic remedies are prepared when the selected agents (herbs and others) for healing are diluted in water and shaken repeatedly. When ready for use, the remedies may only contain a few molecules of the original agents.

The main principle within homeopathy is known as the law of similars, which states that a substance that can produce symptoms in a healthy person can stimulate the self-healing systems in a sick person with similar symptoms. For example, someone suffering from a cold or hay fever with symptoms of burning, watery eyes, and nasal discharge might be treated with a remedy known as allium cepa or onion, a substance known to make the eyes burn and the nose run. A person suffering from insomnia due to the agitation of an overactive mind might be treated with the remedy coffea cruda, which produces those symptoms in a normal, healthy person. Like cures like.

Like Ayurvedic medicine, homeopathy looks at individuals rather than at diseases. Each of us may suffer a cold in our own unique way. Conventional medicine assumes that all colds are alike and will prescribe a different drug to control each symptom: one for a stuffy nose, one for a sore throat, one for sneezing, and one for achiness.

By contrast, the homeopathic practitioner seeks to discover the unique features of that particular cold. On which side is the sore throat located? What are the characteristics of the discharge in amount, color, and consistency? Does the cold move to the sinuses or chest? What were the causative factors that contributed to the onset of the illness: stress, fatigue, anger, lack of sleep, exposure to climate changes? The homeopath then chooses the remedy that matches these unique symptoms in order to stimulate the body's own self-healing systems to respond.

The idea that water and only a few molecules can achieve results is what disturbs the scientists who debunk homeopathy; they can't believe that so little of a healing agent is in the remedy. If water has a memory, though, then it's certainly possible that the needed energy signature for the healing is still within the diluted remedy.

In the early 1980s, Jacques Benveniste, a noted French physician, allergist, and researcher served as head of the French National Institute for Health and Medical Research. One of his lab assistants accidentally diluted a solution of antigens too much, having misread some instructions. The actual concentration of the medicine was much lower than it should have been. Nevertheless it worked just fine for the patient. Another doctor in the practice, who was also a homeopath by training, realized that this lab technician had inadvertently proved a basic principle of homeopathy: that the lower the concentration of the active substance, the stronger the effect: less is more.

Deeper connections

The idea that less is more is common in Western medicine. When radiation therapy first began, much higher concentrations were used, with side-effects reported. In time, much safer levels were prescribed that worked as well or better. With vaccines, the whole idea was to take a tiny amount of the causative agent and let the body learn how to resist it.

After discovering the mistake, the lab continued testing along the same lines, diluting the active ingredient more and more. When they got to a certain dilution level, the positive effect of the treatment spiked markedly. Yet strangely enough, at this point of dilution, there was virtually no measurable trace of the active ingredient left in the solution! Barely a few molecules remained. This is exactly what homeopaths would have predicted: the weaker the dilution, the more powerful the effect. This process was replicated in labs in four different countries with the same results, which were published in *Nature*, a prestigious professional journal.

You can imagine the uproar that caused in the popular press and the scientific community. How could *Nature* publish an article about the nonsensical idea that water could retain the "memory" of the effective molecules of the healing agent?

Soon afterward, a group of scientists arrived at the lab, along with a professional skeptic. The experiment was repeated and it worked again. Then the group changed the protocol (the specific steps, rules, and guidelines that define and govern a scientific experiment) and didn't get the same result. Dr. Benveniste's reputation was damaged, with many thinking he had faked the original results. Over a decade later, four other labs replicated the earlier results in double-blind experiments and the doctor was vindicated.

There are a number of reasons why the second experiment by the scientific team might have failed. They changed the protocols, which is like changing the rules of a sport in the middle of the game. Additionally, considering what we know about water and the effect of positive and negative energy, it's very possible that the very thoughts of the super-skeptical team might have influenced the experiment. Dr. Puharich's expression, *mentation affects experimentation,* is especially true in the quantum world of subtle energies. The mind can affect the results.

Homeopathy is in very active use around the world and many attest to its results. Some remarkable healings have taken place using its remedies in a wide range of conditions, from first-aid and self-limiting conditions to more serious complaints.

Drawing Energy from a Plant Directly

The key with many systems involving plants and herbs is to first choose the property that has the right energy signature. Many systems developed techniques to tap into that energy frequency.

Here's a case that took on a more direct approach. In 1965, H. I. Sober, my master teacher in martial arts and energy control, was in the hospital suffering with toxic megacolon, a life-threatening intestinal condition. He was a young man at the time. His Grandmaster teacher came to his bedside, very upset with him. "They tell me this disease is caused, in part, by the mind, and that it has a large psychogenic component. Is that true?" When Sober told him it was, his teacher rebuked him and said, "Do you know who you are?" He challenged him to use the techniques of mind, energy, and spirit he had learned and mastered in the martial arts to heal himself, to use this meditative power to fight against the disease. In the pain of the disease, it seemed he had forgotten that critical mind-energy lesson.

Later that day, Sober reached out with his weakened arm to a plant that someone had brought to the hospital. He held it and mentally drew the energy-life from the plant, which withered in his hand. He borrowed its energy, transformed it, and used it to survive.

Shattering Stones and Preconceptions

Master H. I. Sober continues to demonstrate energy techniques rarely seen in the West. Imagine vibrating your fingertips into a 4-inch-thick piece of macadam from a demolition site and literally having it explode into 15 or 20 pieces, or softly tapping a large slab of stone from a riverbed and having it shatter without any hard force. Yet this Grand Master and tenured professor of language and history at Yeshiva University, now in his late 60s, who was told he wouldn't live past the age of 25, still demonstrates these incredible energy phenomena.

Water

Food, herbs, and remedies all are part of what we naturally utilize to heal ourselves. Throughout history, though, there has been an even more prevalent healing tool. From ancient times, water has been used for purposes of purification and cleansing.

Charging Water for Energy Healing

Healers in many cultures have energized water with their hands. In all likelihood, many herbal and homeopathic remedies have become more effective after the healer's hands left a memory imprint on the water molecules.

You may remember the healer Oscar Estabany from his work with the founders of therapeutic touch in Chapter 7. In one classic case, Estabany treated sealed bottles of water by holding them in his hands for 15 or 20 minutes. The water was then used in double-blind experiments to treat new barley seeds. The plants that were watered with his "treated" water grew two or three times healthier, bigger, and stronger than the ones in the control group.

Of Mice and Enzymes

MISC.

In addition to being a powerful healer of human patients, Estabany was renowned for working on horses in the Hungarian cavalry. He was also one of the most lab-tested healers in recent times. Research in the 1960's showed that mice who had a portion of skin removed were healed significantly faster by Estabany's treatment than the wounded mice who were not treated by him. In other studies, he was repeatedly able to stimulate the activity of the enzyme trypsin as measured on a known substrate in vitro.

Dr. Puharich spent a good deal of time measuring the E.L.F. frequencies put out by water that had been treated by healers like Israel Carmel, an Israeli healer. Carmel would routinely give patients water he had treated with his hands and reported great success. Puharich determined that the frequency of 8 hz was present and dominant in all the samples of Carmel's treated water.

All this research by Puharich was done inside his Faraday cage, an all-copper room that screened out radio and electromagnetic waves. Only the E.L.F. got through, making it an ideal place for measuring and enhancing healing and psychic energies. It was amazing to see the effects of energy on water, clearly depicted on battery-operated oscilloscopes, digital counters, and other high-tech measurement devices.

Some energy healers working with patients from out of town will send a sealed bottle of water that they've charged with their hands, exclusively for the patient's use. When I've used water this way, I first have patients practice breathing and centering exercises, then take a tablespoon of the treated water, mix it with a full glass of filtered water, and drink it slowly and reverently. The charged water can have a positive effect, but, in addition, the patients bring their own healing energy to the water by their preparation, and by drinking it in a healing frame of mind, making the effect that much greater.

Why Faraday Cages

The reason that research in extra-sensory perception is often conducted inside a Faraday cage is that radio and electromagnetic signals are blocked when the room is sealed. All the technology inside the Faraday cage to do the measuring and recording has to be battery-operated; the 60 hz wires of normal electric lines would interfere with subtle energy measurements.

Living Water for Energy Healing

Many cultures believed water to have mystical properties. In the Jewish tradition, for example, a *mikvah,* or a body of living water, was used to cleanse both people and objects of ritual impurities. It was what John the Baptist was doing in pre-Christian days.

Living water refers to water from springs, wells, or natural bodies such as oceans and lakes. A **mikvah** can also refer to a man-made structure, as long as the water within it is in direct contact with living rainwater. Mikvahs are used for purifying people or objects from ritual impurity and for performing conversions.

Because mikvah water is traditionally associated with healing and cleansing, Puharich and I conducted the following experiment to see if there was a scientific basis for this.

Two identical bottles were filled with water, one with mikvah water, the other with plain tap water. To maintain a control, the bottles were only handled by individuals who knew nothing about a mikvah or the experiment.

When the two bottles were measured in the Faraday cage, the mikvah water measured at exactly 8 hz, the heartbeat of the earth and the ideal brain wave for healing. The control sample wasn't even close, with numbers bouncing all over the place on the digital counter.

Essential Takeaways

- Macrobiotics use certain types of food and methods of eating to help balance the energy matrix.

- Ayurvedic medicine, a complete and complex system of energy healing, has found a new life in the West after thousands of years.

- Homeopathy utilizes the energy signatures of plants and herbs to create diluted remedies that work in a like-heals-like approach.

- Whether it's charged by a healer or shaken and diluted in a homeopathic remedy, water continues to be one of the most utilized tools to enhance and extend energy healing.

chapter 11

Remote-View Energy Healing

Tuning into the energy matrix at a distance

Remote viewing and astral travel

Power-packing another healer

Case studies, from basic to mind-blowing

All the systems of energy healing we have discussed so far have one thing in common: they're done with the healer and the patient touching or being very close to one another. Remote-view healing is when a healer is able to diagnose and treat a patient from a distance, without any physical contact, and more than just a few inches away.

Background and Variations of Remote Viewing

There are two things taking place in remote-view healing, also referred to as non-local healing. First, the healer tunes in to a patient's energy matrix at a distance. Second, the healer downloads or uploads healing information.

Once you accept the underlying principle of energy healing—that people have a discrete energy signature that is as unique as their fingerprint—then tuning into the frequency of that signature shouldn't be any more difficult when the patient is physically in the room or many miles away. You can place a cell phone call to a friend across the street or across the planet; as long as you can get a signal, they sound exactly the same.

As far as downloading diagnostic information and uploading healing energy, we've learned that E.L.F. scalar waves are nonattenuating, meaning that they don't weaken over distance. By that same logic, once you accept the idea that healers can accomplish a healing dialogue with a patient locally, the strength of the energy shouldn't be diminished over a greater distance.

The greatest challenge in remote healing is the additional burden on the healer to maintain concentration without the patient's body being there. In local healing (when you're in the same room as the patient), if your eyes are closed and your mind starts to wander, you can open your eyes and look at the patient to bring your attention back to the healing. It's not as simple for most people to re-focus when the patient isn't in the room.

Remote Viewing or Out-of-Body

When discussing remote healing, people often wonder whether the healer's energy matrix is actually traveling to the patient's location or just viewing the patient from a distance. The former is usually called *out-of-body travel* or an out-of-body experience (or astral travel), and implies that some part of the healer (a mobile center of consciousness) is actually leaving the physical body and going somewhere else.

Finding Meaning

Out-of-body travel is when an energy aspect of the healer (the energy matrix in our common vocabulary, but also called the astral or etheric body) is able to leave the body and travel elsewhere. The healer remains tethered to the body by a so-called silver-blue cord but is also conscious at the remote site.

By contrast, remote viewing, sometimes called mind travel, implies that the healer's energy matrix stays where it is while he or she opens a kind of energy "Skype" connection and, through mind action, senses the patient from a distance.

As to which form of remote healing is taking place, we can't ever really be sure. If you dream that you're flying, does that mean you have left your body and are actually flying in some energy or spirit form? Or does it mean that some part of your brain took an imagined flight and turned it into a more sensory experience? No one knows. Your report of the experience is completely subjective.

Peter Hurkos, a famous psychic who worked on many police cases and government projects, said he saw a screen in his mind when he was "on." He was able to view things at great distances with incredible detail but didn't believe he ever left his body's location.

It may surprise you to know that Helen Keller, in addition to her amazing sensory skills that compensated for her lost sight and hearing, was also quite psychic. She and Greta were close friends, and at one visit, Helen said, "You must excuse me a moment" and slumped in her chair, motionless. Two minutes later she snapped upright. Greta asked her what happened. Helen replied, "I've been to the Alps," and proceeded to describe her visit for almost an hour. She believed that she'd had an astral or out-of-body experience that was, to her, quite real.

Regardless of whether this travel is real on an energy level or just imaginary, the human mind seems to have the ability to experience things and encounter people at a great distance. Silva Mind Method, Reiki, and Therapeutic Touch all have techniques for remote viewing and remote-view healing.

Edgar Cayce

One of the people responsible for bringing the idea of remote-view healing to the modern arena is Edgar Cayce (pronounced *KAY-see*). Known as the "sleeping prophet," he was able to enter a trance state and, with only the name of the subject, provide diagnosis and suggest treatment for thousands of patients. He had the amazing ability to find someone with just a name. Most of Cayce's readings were about health, although he covered many other subjects as well. Though he died in 1945, many of his healing suggestions—or "prescriptions"—are still studied today.

Cayce Massage Technique

Dr. Harold J. Reilly developed a system of whole-body massage based entirely on principles and techniques channeled by Cayce. Cayce massage is one of the most powerful full-body massages you can experience. Recipients of these massages claim they can feel energy moving, almost flying, all over their bodies during and after the massage.

The WEB and the Energy Matrix in Remote Viewing

To understand what happens in remote healing, let's briefly review our working theory of what happens during local energy healing. The healer enters a meditative state and gets in touch with his energy matrix, which should be as grounded as possible. After much practice and meditative discipline, the healer has been able to upgrade his energy matrix to the point where the chakras, the nerve plexuses of his matrix, are operating at a very high level of efficiency. This upgraded energy matrix is now able to efficiently draw from the energy battery of the planet and from the WEB's energy that fills the universe.

When the healer is ready, he begins by preparing the patient for energy healing, utilizing guided speech, breathing, music, or some other process to assist the patient in receiving energy healing and getting in touch with her own energy matrix.

The two energy matrices phase-lock, or achieve radio-communication with one another. The patient's energy matrix's information is now accessible to the healer, enabling him to download information about the source of the problem and how best to fix it.

All of this occurs in remote healing as well, the only difference being that the healer doesn't have the benefit of proximity. As we've already learned, your energy matrix contains your entire personal energy history, even if your conscious mind can't access it. To take it one step further, the WEB, the worldwide energy bubble, has the energy history of the universe, of all the energy matrices that have ever existed. So with the proper focus, a healer can log on to the WEB and download information from an energy matrix on the other side of the world, much the way we can log on to the internet and see a web video posted by someone far away. You just need to know the right URL address or, in this case, the individual energy signature.

The Akashic Record

In Indian cultures, the universal energy database is called the Akashic record; yogis and mystics have always claimed that it's possible to learn to access this database. They report that all the knowledge in the universe is stored in the Akashic record. If one's energy matrix is evolved enough, it will have access to advanced knowledge about healing and spiritual growth. That may seem far out, but it's not that different from how we access our own global information database every day by logging on to the internet!

Whether the healer and patient are touching or thousands of miles apart, the basics of energy healing are the same. It's considered remote if the healer can't physically touch the patient, whether they're on opposite sides of the planet or opposite sides of a room.

Focus and Power-Packing in Remote Healing

One of the most important necessities for remote healing is the ability to focus the mind and hold it there. Someone experienced in meditation shouldn't have difficulty doing this; it may not be so simple for a novice. If you can imagine someone clearly and distinctly in your mind, you have already overcome the greatest hurdle. Many healers prefer to have a picture of the patient. Some prefer to hold an object belonging to the patient in their hands. This helps them tune in to the energy signature of the patient's energy matrix.

Another very helpful adjunct to remote healing is to have a group of grounded healers working on the healing with you. The primary healer is the one who can phase-lock most easily with the remote patient. The others are there to help anchor the healer while she's in the session, and to provide her with as much energy as necessary to accomplish the goal of the healing. Ideally, the power-pack should be comprised of trained healers or, at the very least, healers in training. They must know how to ground themselves (see Chapter 14) and how to transmit energy to the healer.

Case Studies in Remote Healing

Basic remote-view healing is no more complicated than healers getting in touch with their grounded energy matrix, phase-locking with the patient's energy matrix, and sending energy to the patient. This has been part of the human experience for millennia. Here are a few cases of remote-view healing, some of them very simple and others that may blow your mind!

Beginner's Luck with Remote-View Healing

It's one thing to be taught about remote healing and quite another to discover that you can do it on your own.

Dr. Andrew Chernick began studying both yoga and karate in the early 1970's. As part of his yoga training, he learned many of the basic RB (Reflex Balance) massage areas. He took to the idea of energy healing massage very quickly.

One night, he was sitting at home in New York watching TV with his wife Raquel, also a student in karate and yoga. He casually crisscrossed his legs over hers on the coffee table in front of the couch then suddenly began to notice that some of the RB points on his feet began to ache. He pulled his feet up to palpate them but discovered that they weren't at all tender, which surprised him.

As they continued to ache, he flashed on the idea that maybe the points that ached on his own feet were actually Raquel's imbalances, which had manifested on his feet through some kind of weird energy wire-crossing interference pattern.

Operating on that hunch, he took her feet and began to massage them. Sure enough, every point he'd felt aching on his feet was tender on hers. The significance of this discovery was that he was able to phase-lock with another person's energy matrix and derive information from it through his own feet, rather than hers. The question that occurred to him was whether he could do this from a distance. So he tested it on a complete stranger, from across a large room. It worked! Essentially, he had discovered an early stage of remote healing, learning to tune in to the vibratory signature of someone else's energy matrix.

Remote Massage

Whenever Greta worked on a remote healing case, her protocol was simple. The patient, wherever she was, would lie still for about 5 or 10 minutes before the pre-scheduled time of the healing, breathing quietly and evenly and preparing to receive the healing energies. Greta would get into a ready state as well, breathing, rooting, and focusing. At the predetermined time, Greta would focus on phase-locking her energy matrix with the patient's while other trained healers gathered around to power-pack. In addition to the many healers she worked with, her husband, Dick, some of their grown children, and I were often part of that pack.

Greta would then try to sense the problem and target whatever energy was needed to balance it. After the session, she would call the patient on the phone and ask what she felt.

stay Grounded

It's very important to make sure that the healer's energy matrix stays grounded during a remote or out-of-body session. Greta felt strongly about having power-pack healers present during remote healings. This kept her safe, especially if she was going out of body.

One night, moments before she was to begin a remote healing, Greta suggested that I do the remote and she would power-pack me. I had no idea what to do. She said to picture the patient lying in front of me and imagine palpating her feet just as I did when she was in the room. I sat with my eyes closed, rotating my thumbs in the air into imaginary feet. To an outside observer, it would have looked pretty weird!

After the session we called the patient and asked her what she felt during the healing. She said, "This healing was a little different than the other remote sessions we've done. I don't know how to describe what I felt except to say that it felt like when Michael massages my feet. The feet were a little achy and tingling just like during the massage. It was pretty strange." We all laughed in amazement. I guess I had done my first remote healing!

From the point of view of the novice, power-packing during a healing, remote or local, is a way for new healers to participate in the beautiful act of healing. If you've begun your training, take every opportunity to work with master healers if you can. The potential for improved skills and personal growth, as well as scoring some great karmic brownie points, makes it a worthwhile experience.

Remote Healing and the Butterfly Ring

In energy healing classes, students are often encouraged to bring friends or family to work on. Only the students know what the patients' problems are, but they don't reveal them until afterward. Whenever Greta joined remotely, she wanted to know as little as possible, preferably only the most general location of the problem.

Dr. Harvey Grossbard, OMD, was a teenager at the time of one such class. This class was his first introduction to energy healing, and he brought a friend with a benign growth on her optic nerve that was causing severe headaches. In this case, we all knew the problem in advance. Because the case was pretty serious, Greta agreed to do a remote healing from Westport, Connecticut. The students formed an energy circle around the patient to help power-pack, Lillian sat at the patient's head with her hands over the patient's eye, and Greta sent energy through Lillian's hands into the patient.

When the session began, the energy was very strong, attributable to all the different energies focused and working together. After the session, Greta said she had no trouble getting to our location but that, unfortunately, something was blocking her view. Some "yellow or gold blurry mass with shiny sparkles on it" was in her way and she couldn't get to the patient's eye. No one understood what could have caused it. Even so, she said she'd sent a powerful burst of energy to the girl's eye.

Lillian suddenly realized exactly what it was: she was wearing a ring with a small gold butterfly with diamond eyes and antennae. It was on the hand that was over the patient's eye during the healing. Why this ring had blocked Greta's line of sight was anyone's guess, but it had. There was a second attempt, sans ring, that was successful: the girl reported seeing a bright flash of light, and her headaches disappeared.

Viewing the Remote Viewer

During the early days of his training, Andrew Chernick was present during many healing sessions. When his father was hospitalized, suffering from *tardive dyskinesia*, Andrew asked me to come upstate to Monticello, New York, to work on him.

Tardive dyskinesia is a neurological disorder in which a patient often experiences continuous involuntary hand and facial movements. The tongue and lips are in continuous motion, appearing to the outsider as if the patient is wildly trying to feed himself.

The night before traveling upstate, I did a remote-view healing, just to tune in to the patient. I rooted and began to visualize Andrew's father, imagining that I was at the foot of his bed palpating his feet.

The next day when I arrived, his father remarked that it was nice to see me again. Andrew and I were confused. I had just arrived, and we'd never met before. But when he thanked me for the massage the night before, and accurately described the clothes I had been wearing while doing the remote massage, I understood. He had actually seen me standing at the foot of his bed doing the RB massage!

It was pretty freaky. I hadn't intended to "travel" anywhere, nor was I aware of having done so. All I did was imagine a man I'd never met and proceed to do my thing. We were all quite blown away by this experience. More importantly, the patient came out of that bout with the disease very nicely.

Essential Takeaways

- In remote-view healing a healer is able to diagnose and treat a patient from a distance, without any physical contact.
- Some healers believe they are traveling out of body to remote locations, while others describe it as viewing the remote location from where they are.

- If a healer can phase-lock her energy matrix with the energy matrix of the patient, it should make no difference how far away the patient's body is located.
- Remote healing increases the importance of healers being able to quiet and aim the mind, sustaining it for a period of time.

Part 3

Healing Others Starts with Healing Yourself

Whether your interest in energy healing is from the vantage point of a potential patient, or of becoming an energy healer yourself, there are basic techniques that you can begin learning right now to help balance your energy matrix and stimulate your body's own self-healing systems.

These include techniques of breathing, centering, and ocular divergence to better engage energy healing, and self-massage to clean out your energy matrix. Finally, I have devoted a chapter to teach some of the basics of sensitizing yourself to the energy fields around you—and in you!

All of these can facilitate self-healing, as well as prepare you to be a more effective energy healer.

chapter 12

Attitudes for Energy Healing

The first—and last—lesson in energy healing

Keeping it light, simple, and selfless

The importance of self-discipline

Skills are easy to teach; attitudes are not. Perhaps because we're so used to the idea of memorizing facts and lists in school, because that's what we're graded on, we don't factor in our attitudinal readiness when we begin to explore a new subject. No one ever asked you how you *feel* about algebra. Your job in math class is to learn how to come up with the right answers. In energy healing, you'll achieve greater success if you start with the right attitude.

DeVries taught that the first lesson in yoga is character. Our character is a reflection of our attitudes and how they manifest in day-to-day living.

Starting with the Right Attitude

Very few people in the West are born into homes that have well-established attitudes about energy healing. In parts of the world where energy healing is the norm— some communities in India, China, and Hawaii, for example—that attitude permeates the home and cultural worldview. I want to share with you some ideas that will help clarify what I believe are some of the essentials for achieving success in the study of energy healing.

For those already involved in energy work, these ideas will probably feel familiar and comfortable. For those just getting started, let me say this: the attitude is the most important thing. I would go so far as to say that a positive attitude is even more important than having natural talent. Anyone can be trained to be a healer—you don't necessarily need to be born with a wondrous gift—but it won't happen if the attitude isn't there.

When I hear about people who were born with amazing abilities, I often wonder how many others might have incredible gifts that are dormant because they haven't been discovered yet. Who knows whether the greatest opera singer in the world would have discovered her gift if she had been born in a community that didn't allow singing? How would she ever know? Just think of the amazing potential within each of us. You might be a potential master of something you've never even dreamed of.

If your heart has brought you to this exploration, you're in the right place. Let's explore some core attitudinal ideas in energy healing.

Y.E.S.

I summarize a simple formula for success in energy healing with the acronym Y.E.S.: Yield, Energize, Sweeten. Simply stated: yield, or let go of the ego and accept a greater body of wisdom; energize by separating yourself meditatively from your material reality and logging on to the WEB; and sweeten reality by sharing some of the energy and light you've brought back.

The Y.E.S. principle is my version of a teaching by Rabbi Israel ben Eliezer, the Ba'al Shem Tov or Master of The Good Name. He was an eighteenth-century practical mystic and the father of the Hassidic movement, a more mystical branch of Jewish Orthodoxy. While the Kabbalistic world wants to bring heaven down to Earth, the Hassidic world wants to bring humanity up to God, a more populist approach.

The principle is very simple, and I've seen it in many versions in a myriad of traditions. Most schools of meditation, inner development, and spiritual growth would agree with the first two of these elements without hesitation. The third seems to be less universal.

We begin the process by yielding. The ego is useful as the mask or face we present to the world. We require an ego to function in the day-to-day world, but it can be a barrier to the selflessness that's necessary for energy healing.

At the same time that we're working on letting go of the ego, we prepare to accept the responsibility or burden of living our lives by a higher set of values. We yield to a source of knowledge greater than ourselves. For some people, this can be a religious calling. For others, it's a philosophical one, like the oath to "do no harm" doctors take. Think of this as the stage in which we prepare the chariot of our energy matrix to log on to the WEB. But it must be done from a posture of yielding.

Because we've achieved the 8 hz brain waves in the first stage, we can utilize our meditative skills to phase-lock with the heartbeat of the earth and log on to the WEB. Our goal in the second stage is to energize our energy matrix and take off to the highest levels of the WEB we can reach. There, we can receive whatever wisdom we're ready for, and download it into our energy matrix, which involves a lot of hard work and time.

When we're prepared we come to the third stage, which is the most important one, in my opinion. Every meditative school in the world will tell you about the first two stages. Many of them are content to reach that level of selflessness in their metaphorical caves in the mountains. But I believe that the real work begins when you come back down to Earth. We have to bring that wisdom down from out there and share it so that the higher energy can be used to sweeten and repair the world. Energy healing is a beautiful and meaningful way to do it.

MISC.

Giving Doesn't Mean Losing

The famous "love professor" and philosopher Leo Buscaglia once said, "If I taught you everything that I know, I'd still know everything that I know!" Well, that's true in healing, too. If I share/channel all the energy I can during a healing, I still have all the energy I had, plus the additional, wonderful feeling of having helped to sweeten someone's life a little.

It's not enough to strive for your own personal body-mind-spirit growth. That can easily make you self-centered and selfish. The goal of the Y.E.S.

principle is to remind us to try to reach for something higher, but with the added commitment to bring that higher light back down into your energy matrix and share it, to leave the world a little better off than when you got here. To quote an ancient Jewish proverb, "You don't have to finish that work, but you're not free to abandon it." That is energy healing at its best.

So remember: just say Y.E.S.!

Keep It Light, Keep It Simple, and Keep the Ego out of It

This is one of my teacher DeVries's favorite sayings, a little teaching that packs an attitudinal guidance punch.

When we say "Keep it light," we mean that we shouldn't take ourselves too seriously. You need to have a sense of humor in—and about—life. DeVries once shared with me the qualities her teacher most liked to see in a student: very serious about his studies but with a grand sense of humor. The balance of the two makes life more livable. Too much of either quality creates an imbalance in life that often leads to excess. Today we're more likely to say, "Lighten up," but "Keep it light" says so much more.

From an energy point of view, it also means you should keep your mind on the fact that all things are light and energy. When you get bogged down with all the craziness of the day, remember that it's all light. Reality isn't as dense as you think; it's not worth getting attached to the material stuff. If it's all energy, you can learn to ground, neutralize, modify, or share it.

Love life, have a sense of humor, and always remember that, because all *is* light, every moment can be an opportunity for energy healing on some level. If you're keeping your mind on the light around you, then even a simple thank-you, as shown by Dr. Emoto's water crystals, might create a positive healing energy in your energy matrix, and in someone else's, too.

Changing the world is tough; healing it, almost impossible. While the world is complicated, its fundamental truths are simple. Anyone who wants to be an energy healer needs to learn all the background, science, philosophy, and skills necessary to do the job and then forget it all; forget the words. Become a chariot of light (an energy matrix), log on to the WEB, and surf it; download some of its high-energy light, bring it back, and get started in your sharing and healing.

But keep it simple. Explore and absorb what you can today. More will be there waiting for you tomorrow. The great truths are simple, though difficult at times to understand and internalize. The old adage "When the student is ready, that master will appear" doesn't necessarily mean you have to wait for a wise, old, bearded teacher to knock on your door; it means that you'll only hear and internalize a lesson when you're ready to.

Keeping the ego out of it is the hardest part of all. Don't get super-proud of your successes; don't get depressed over what seem to be failures. You'll find success much sooner if you keep all that other pride/depression junk out of the way. Sometimes you may come upon that state of selflessness with ease; sometimes you may struggle in frustration because nothing seems to be happening.

When you do a random act of kindness with no ego involved, you feel good about yourself, and so the ego swells up to take credit for it. It's a catch-22. Staying humble and selfless requires continual vigilance on your part. Remember this mantra: keep it light, keep it simple, and keep the ego out of it!

Reaching the Peek

Occasionally, the cosmos might give you a preview, a small peek at what lies ahead if you can achieve that state of selflessness so important in the healing process. I'll share an example from one of the most profound moments of my life.

Years ago I had the occasion to tell DeVries about an experience I had when I was 17: I was a counselor at a sleep-away camp in the Catskill Mountains in upstate New York. One night, after lights out, I couldn't sleep. So I went for a walk down by the dammed-up creek where the kids would swim. There was no moon out and no bothersome electric lights nearby. It seemed as if every star in the Milky Way was visible. I lay back in the thick grass, feeling the first dew on my back, just watching the stars. I noticed a very large bright one in the center of the sky. Maybe it was a planet … I don't know. I started playing tricks with my eyes. I would stare at the star without blinking for so long that all the other stars seemed to blur and disappear. Then I blinked, and they all came back.

Then I suddenly stood up and reached out for that star with my right hand, fingers spread, palm diagonally upward. I didn't really think about what I was doing; I just did it. As I kept my eyes on the star, I suddenly became overwhelmed with the thought of how tiny my hand was. And not just my hand; my body, the ground, the planet, everything was so tiny. Earth was just a tiny speck in a galaxy of a hundred billion stars. And *that* galaxy was just a speck in a universe of over a hundred billion galaxies. And there was my tiny speck of a hand against the star-filled sky. I had a profound sense of being tiny ... of being *nothing* against this incredible backdrop of the heavens.

And then something happened. It was so abrupt it almost seemed to click. I was no longer infinitesimally small. I was the whole universe. I was the stars and the galaxies and the heavens and the earth. I was overwhelmed with the oneness and love that seemed to surround and embrace me. I have no idea how long I stood there with my hand up reaching for the star. There was no sense of my arm tiring. I just stood there, at one with all there is.

Slowly the sensation began to fade, but there was no sadness. I knew that the power of this moment would never leave me completely. Even as I write this, it's like I'm experiencing it again right now.

I knew I had to do it again, so the next night I went back and followed the exact same steps: lying in the grass, reaching to the star, standing ... and standing ... but nothing happened that night. Or the next. Or the one after that. But I knew that I was going to do whatever it took to get that feeling—if you can even call it a feeling; it was so much more than that—back again.

stay Grounded

When something amazing happens to you, you feel empowered, as if you'd done something to make it happen. Don't get carried away! Keep the ego out of it and yield to the higher intelligence that guided you to that moment. You're a part of the universe, not its center!

As I finished telling the story, DeVries smiled and said, "You had a peek experience." I agreed, thinking she meant that it was a peak, or a natural high. But she said, "No, you misunderstand. I mean a peek experience; p-e-e-k, not p-e-a-k; nature gave you a peek into her mysteries. If you want to see more, you'll have to earn it. By achieving the kind of controlled discipline of body and mind that your yoga and martial arts encourage, you will earn the right to touch nature's wonders on your own terms."

This peek into the mysteries of nature, infinite oneness, whatever you want to call it, helped me focus and has guided my life ever since. I came to realize that it didn't work the second night, or the many nights thereafter, because I wanted to be part of the whole without being small first. I wanted to energize without yielding. And the irony was that my ego, having experienced it the first night, couldn't become small enough to let it happen again because it was too bloated with pride over an achievement I hadn't caused anyway.

The Importance of Self-Discipline

If you'd ever been in one of my classes, you would have heard me tell the following story about discipline.

One day a student brought in a flyer she'd seen on the wall at the Center for Psychological Services at Wake Forest University. It read: "Discipline is remembering what you want!" She thought I would really like it because of my strong emphasis on disciplining oneself for both physical health and mental centeredness. I looked at it, thought about it, and almost immediately said that I didn't care for it. Somewhat hurt, I think, she asked why. I said, "Because discipline is remembering what you want *and doing something about it.*" Remembering is fine. I may remember that I want to exercise today, to do my breathing drills, to center, to meditate, to pray. But I don't really get any points unless I *do* something. Remembering isn't enough.

But that's only half the story of discipline. For your discipline to be effective long term, you must have both patience and perseverance as balancing elements. DeVries began teaching that lesson about the balance of discipline and patience on my first day of class.

I had been studying yoga with Greta for eight years when I became a First-Degree Black Belt. In honor of the occasion, she gave me a gift that would forever change my life: my first class with DeVries. I was very nervous. I stepped on the mat and, after going through some basic warm-up postures, she asked me to go into a headstand. The mat was a little spongier than the one I practiced on regularly, so I bobbled a bit, got my balance, and continued to go up into the posture. DeVries stopped me and asked me to come down. She saw the disappointment on my face and looked deeply into my eyes with loving firmness. She said, "Andron, always remember that the first and last lesson in yoga is character, not posture."

"Don't be disappointed about the headstand," she continued. "You'll only need to develop greater control and movement from your center. That will take some time and a great deal of patience. That's what it's all about: practice in peace, with patience and perseverance." As she continued to talk, this 80-plus-year-old Grand Master lowered her head to the mat and floated upward, as smoothly as a wisp of smoke, into a headstand and continued to move through a series of different inverted postures with her legs and body. She then folded her legs into a *lotus* posture and after a moment floated back down, in slow motion, to a sitting position. She landed in perfect control and silence. It was the most breathtaking movement I had ever seen. As she continued to speak to me gently throughout the demonstration, her breath, even the tenor of her voice, never changed.

Finding
Meaning

Lotus is the king of sitting meditative postures. The legs are tied in a knot, with each of the feet resting on the opposite thigh, resembling a lotus blossom. The pose is hard enough, but getting into it effortlessly, without using your hands, upside down, is exceedingly difficult.

When I got my breath back from that amazing demonstration, I said, "It's going to take a lot of practice to ever do that. But practice makes perfect, right?" She responded, "No, practice does not make perfect. Practice makes *permanent*! Be sure you learn it correctly first. Then practicing it correctly will make it perfect."

I didn't care how long it was going to take me. I was going to learn to do that! And for 10 more years, until her death, I studied with DeVries as a student and, later, as a teacher-trainee.

Over the years I've been fortunate enough to study with some of the finest teachers the world has to offer, in subjects as diverse as t'ai chi ch'uan, yoga, healing, science, Kabbalah, and theater. In their own particular paradigms, they each taught about living and loving, character and discipline. They taught me, guided me, badgered me, "beat" me, broke me, and helped put me back together. When I look back at some of the lessons I've developed over the years, I find they're all based on the foundations laid by those teachers.

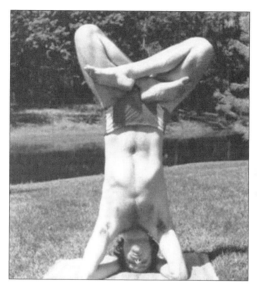

The author's lotus headstand.

Beginning Each Day

Each morning, as a sort of wake-up exercise, DeVries instructed me to raise my arms above my head, make a very tight fist, and fan my fingers outward, one at a time, as if each finger was reaching to infinity. It's a great little exercise that improves flexibility and circulation in the fingers, something most people tend to lose as they age.

As we practiced this at the beginning of a yoga class, though, DeVries would say a simple five-line poem, or mantra, if you will, as each finger spread out from the fist. I love those lines, and the exercise, and have repeated them daily for over 40 years.

> *Each Day, say thank you for being alive*
>
> *Each Day, take responsibility for your physical performance*

Each Day, take responsibility for your mental performance

Each Day, be careful of human nature

Each Day, behold the wonder of Mother Nature

The idea of beginning each day by giving thanks is nothing new. Most religions have such prayers in their morning liturgy. From an energy standpoint, though, we can take it to a whole new level. Just think of Dr. Emoto's water crystals and the profound impact two words like thank you can have on your water-based body, as well as your energy matrix. Imagine yourself at the base of Jacob's ladder. Log on to the WEB and send your message of thanks up the ladder. As you do, extend your thumb outward in the stretch.

The second and third lines, taking responsibility for your physical and mental performance, are interesting in their word choice. The simple meaning is that you should discipline yourself to do the daily breathing and exercise plans you've undertaken. In addition, be sure to practice the mental part: quieting the mind, centering, rooting, meditating, praying, or whatever your mental discipline is.

What strikes me is the use of the word performance. As I say that line each morning, I focus on the idea that it's not enough to just do the physical and mental work (yield and energize). I want to bring the inner benefit of that work with me out into the world and operate from that place all day (share/sweeten). It's not enough to meditate morning and night and then be harried and uncentered all day. The purpose is to incorporate that meditative center into your whole day.

deeper connections

One of the hardest things for a stage actor to do is say the same thing over and over again, first in rehearsal and then in performance. To make the words feel fresh and new, you have to imagine you're saying them for the first time every time. Then your acting achieves the quality of living truthfully. Try to think about that when you say any personal prayer or mantra. Saying it each morning as if you've never said it before will change your day.

The fourth line, "Be careful of human nature," alerts you to the idea that other people aren't necessarily operating from the same paradigm as you are. Try to engage them at their own level, whether that's higher or lower than your own. If they're higher, aspire upward. If they're lower, be patient and understanding. That's even more important if you're coming together for energy healing. You can't phase-lock with the patient if you're on two different frequencies.

In addition, be careful of your own human nature. All of us, at some moments, can be operating from a place we might not be proud of later. Sure, by all means, be careful of others' poor behavior, but first and last, be careful of your own. If you're not working, from the very best part of you, try to be aware of that and fix it through self-reflection, contemplation, and preparation before you enter a healing session. It's like that old saying: [Energy] Physician: heal thyself!

Finally, as you stretch and roll that last finger out into a completely open hand, try to embrace something bigger than yourself. Behold the wonder of creation, of the WEB that surrounds our universe. If you come from a specific religious tradition, many prayers with this exact theme may come to mind. I especially like to do the last line while looking out the window and reflecting on some aspect of nature, or even repeating the whole exercise outside. It's a beautiful way to start each day.

DeVries's poem is a great complement to the famous 12-line poem that is thought (or said) in yoga while performing the Sun Salutation exercise:

> *Look to this day!*
>
> *For it is life, the very life of life.*
>
> *In its brief course lie all the verities and realities of existence.*
>
> *The bliss of growth,*
>
> *The glory of action,*
>
> *The splendor of beauty.*
>
> *For yesterday is already a dream*
>
> *And tomorrow is only a vision.*

But today, well-lived, make every yesterday a dream of happiness

And every tomorrow, a vision of hope.

Look well, therefore, to this day.

Such is the salutation to the dawn.

A Final Thought on Attitude and Discipline

We've explored attitude as well as discipline. Which is more important? Simply put, both. You can't have a dreamy vision without the discipline to bring the dream to reality. And you can't just do the working out without some vision of what you want to achieve.

Your own personal objective could be any number of things—improved physical health or better stress management. It could be upgrading the power of your energy matrix so you can log on to the WEB and achieve a higher state of awareness. That's a decision you have to make (if you haven't already) for yourself. But whatever you choose, practice in peace, with patience and perseverance.

Essential Takeaways

- Y.E.S. is a guiding principle to help you keep on track as you study energy healing.
- Keep it light, keep it simple, and keep the ego out of it. That says it all.
- Discipline isn't just remembering what you want. It's remembering what you want and doing something about it.
- Take some time each day to reflect on yourself and on your world.

chapter 13

Breathing

The power of breathing in energy healing

The rules and mechanics of effective breath-work

Breathing skills to charge and calm the energy matrix

You need food, water, and oxygen to survive. You can live without water for a few days and food for a few weeks, but without air, you can't live for more than a few minutes! Considering how critical our respiratory system is to our survival, it's amazing how little time we spend thinking about it. We're constantly thinking about our diet or whether we're drinking enough water, but we tend to forget about our breathing, other than occasionally reminding ourselves to take a deep breath when we're feeling nervous.

Breathing—and specifically controlled breathing—can have a profound impact on our general health, as well as our effectiveness in energy healing.

Breath-Work

Of all the various things I've studied and practiced—yoga, meditation, martial arts, even theater (which involves projecting from the diaphragm)—the single-greatest common denominator is breathing. Each of these disciplines has its own distinct style of breathing to help reach maximum potential. A change in our breathing can help us run faster, punch harder, even sing higher notes. Manipulating our breathing is a way for us to tap into so much potential. Let's take a closer look at the background, rules, and mechanics of breath-work.

Background

Try this simple experiment: Listen carefully for the most distant sound you can hear. It could be a bird, the wind, or a creaky plank in the floor. Listen with as much concentration as you can. Stop reading and do it now.

Did you notice that while you were concentrating on the sound, you stopped breathing entirely? You held your breath for the few seconds it took to do the exercise. The same thing happens when you bang your shin against a chair and grab the painful spot. Or when you concentrate on drawing a very straight line, or try to lift something very heavy. When the mind is concentrating, the breath is automatically suspended. Of course you can override this command, but the automatic response is to hold your breath.

This phenomenon led ancient masters to an idea that is simple and yet profound: if the breath is controlled by the mind, then by learning to control the breath, we can learn to control the mind. A multitude of techniques were developed to test this theory, and the hypothesis soon proved to be true. The masters continued to develop techniques for every eventuality and every state of mind, including breaths to help achieve the highest states of consciousness. They had discovered the link between body and mind—it was the breath.

In fact, the very words that were chosen to describe energy in these ancient cultures are, more often than not, words for breath. Prana, Qi/Chi, and Ki are all terms that mean breath. Most of them are also used to mean spirit and life force as well. In Hebrew, the words for the three basic levels of the *soul* are neh'fesh, ru'ah, and nih'shah'mah, all having to do with the stages of breathing: breathing out, the breath itself, and breathing in.

Deeper connections

Consciousness is like a kite, breath the string that guides it: this Sanskrit saying emphasizes that if your goal is to control the mind, you must first discipline the breath. It's when you try to quiet your mind that you notice how it tends to jump around a lot. By counting the seconds of each inhalation and exhalation, you aim the mind toward a specific target and keep it from wandering. That's the first step toward controlling it.

Discoveries were also made that certain types of controlled breathing might have a profound impact on the physical body, not just the mind or soul. For example, when your diaphragm, the muscle of breath, moves up and down rhythmically, your abdominal organs and glands are given a gentle massage that aids your digestion and calms your emotional state. That's because breathing affects the adrenal glands, the thyroid, and the rectal plexus, all of which are intimately associated with stress and how we handle it.

In Chapter 4, you learned that one of the immediate signs of the fight-or-flight response is accelerated breathing. The opposite is true in the relaxation response: your breath slows down. So by intentionally slowing down the breathing rate, we convince the autonomic nervous system (which doesn't know the difference between real and imaginary stressors), that we're relaxed, thereby short-circuiting an inappropriate evoking of the fight-or-flight response. Sometimes if we need to perform a demanding task, controlled, high-speed breathing can evoke a simulated fight-or-flight response to provide us with the energy needed. By practicing a routine that includes fast then slow breathing, we, in effect, give a workout and attunement to our autonomic nervous system.

Even more basic is the fact that of all the functions in the body that are affected by age, the ones involving breathing have the highest average decreases. Useful lung volume and maximum breathing capacity decrease the most as we age, even more than velocity of nerve-signal transmission, kidney-filtration rate, or pumping efficiency of the heart.

Inspired Breathing

The Latin word for *I breathe* is *spiro*. When we take in something that raises our breath/spirit, we are *in-spired*. When we die, and breathe out our last breath, we are said to *ex-(s)pire*. When our whole body breathes through the skin to keep the body at a stable temperature, we *per-spire*. When people get together and make big plans together, they *con-spire*.

However you look at it, breath and life and spirit are all tied together. The old masters maintained that when air was breathed in, life energy was breathed in as well. The exact nature of this energy may remain unclear, but we certainly have uncovered part of the secret. One of the elements to feeling wonderful and energized is the presence of negative ions on the surface of the body's blood cells. When only positive charges are there, we feel tired, sour, and drained—an effect notoriously associated with the Khamsin winds that plague the Middle East. The Khamsin is a positive ion storm that affects the electrical charge of the body's cells.

On the other hand, technological negative ion generators give us an immediate pick-me-up. We feel alert, refreshed, and quite stimulated. Operating rooms in hospitals and jet airplanes have negative ion generators in them. Research has shown that pilots, surgeons, office workers, and even psychics consistently perform better in a high negative ion environment.

What most people don't realize is that we have negative ion generators right in our own bodies: the heart and the respiratory system. As the blood goes through the heart, the spiral muscles break away negative ions from the oxygen atoms. The heart, in addition to being a blood pump, is a negative ion pump, and its function, in conjunction with specific breathing practices, is to supply every blood cell with a negative surface charge to create a sense of overall wellness.

Why do we feel so good under the influence of negative ions in our bloodstream? Because when the surface of the blood cells is negatively charged, they repel each other like little magnets. As a result they don't clump together, and the oxygen those cells are carrying is more easily absorbed by the body. However, because opposites attract, when antibodies with positive charges on their surface appear on the scene, the positive and negative charges attract each other and the cells can clump together. Oxygen becomes less accessible and we feel tired and weak.

When we practice certain yoga breathing techniques, the increased speed of the breath increases the heart rate. That pushes the blood through the chambers of the heart more quickly, causing the surface electrons of the oxygen atoms to break off in greater numbers. These small, negatively charged electrons are the negative ions.

Negatives as Positives

MISC.

Negative ions are one of the reasons you feel so refreshed in a pine forest, by the seashore, and near waterfalls. Pointed pine needles cause a higher concentration of negative ions to break off as the trees "exhale" oxygen. The rapid motion of the water in a waterfall and the waves breaking against the rocky reefs do exactly the same thing: they break off the electrons from the atoms, which become negative ions. The naturally high level of negative ions at these locations explains why they make us feel so good.

All this talk of energy and ions may seem a little esoteric. Here's a more basic example of the power of controlled breathing. Years ago, while I was teaching a Karate class, I walked around the room watching each student doing his or her Kata (form). I began to listen to their breathing and noticed something I never had before: I could almost tell what rank the student was just by listening to his breath.

This was remarkable, because the first lesson each student learns on the very first day as a white belt beginner is how to do abdominal breathing. Nevertheless, it seemed as if the extent to which they had internalized the ability to transmit energy (power) was directly linked to their capacity to properly breathe with depth. Their breath got better, so their energy transference improved, their forms got stronger, and they were awarded higher belts.

And even though it's something that's taught on the first day, it takes time for students to get it. I started using this concept as a sort of technique therapy: when I can help a student see and hear the differences in their own breathing, it accelerates their development.

Rules

Rather than learning many different breaths, it's much more useful to learn a few and to perform them properly. Before you begin, it's a good idea to keep the following points in mind. You can also find links to helpful videos in the Resources appendix.

1. Refrain from doing too much controlled breathing until your body learns to adjust to the different levels of oxygen and CO_2 in your system; you could become lightheaded. Start gradually and don't increase repetitions beyond a few minutes without the guidance of an experienced teacher. But be careful; there are many qualified teachers who go to extremes too soon rather than choosing a more gradual path.

2. When you inhale, the breath should be drawn in through the nose, not the mouth. This will clean the air as it passes through the little filtering hairs or cilia in your nose, warm the air as it travels the longer path from nose to lungs, and charge the air as it passes the magnet of the sphenoid sinus. One of the only exceptions to nose inhalation is the *bellows breath* in yoga.

> **Finding Meaning**
>
> The **bellows breath** is a rapid breathing technique to charge up the system. You may have learned variations of it in childbirth classes to deal with the pain of contractions. The inhalation, in its most common variation, is done through the mouth, which is okay because it's a shallow breath and the colder air doesn't reach the lungs before it's immediately exhaled.

3. When you exhale for these breaths, breathe out of the mouth, with the "hah" sound. Don't say the word "hah"; whisper it steadily from the back of your throat as you exhale. What about cleaning, warming, and charging the air? That's important when you're bringing dirtier and cooler air into your 98.6°F bodies, but it isn't necessary when you're exhaling toxic air. As a matter of fact, getting the excess CO_2 out of your lungs faster, and not running it through the filter of your nose, makes a lot of sense.

4. Flare your nostrils as you inhale. As the air passes through the nose, try to draw it down and back toward the back of your throat, rather than upward into the sinus cavity. This will increase the amount of air that can be taken in and will gradually increase lung capacity. As you inhale, imagine that you're trying to inhale the fumes of a cough lozenge; you want to get that eucalyptus vapor back and down into the throat. That's the difference between back-and-down breathing and upward breathing. In men, the upward movement of the Adam's apple and tightening of the throat will indicate that the breathing pattern is wrong. There should be no tension in the throat for men or women. Also, in back-and-down breathing, the nostrils flare slightly; in upward breathing, the nostrils close toward each other as if you smelled something bad. It's nature telling you how to breathe effectively.

5. Try to keep the spine erect and body movement minimal during breathing practice.

6. Keep the eyes open at all times to prevent hyperventilation and dizziness. You live with your eyes open; practice breathing with your eyes open.

Mechanics

Before you can learn the three breaths in this chapter, you need to understand the basic mechanics of breathing. It will help to sit by a mirror as you practice these exercises, one that's large enough for you to see your whole torso.

Your two lungs are like big balloons with divided sections known as lobes, three lobes on the right side and two on the left. When you inhale, the lobes are filled with air and expand. When you exhale, the air is forced out and the lungs contract.

But how does it happen? There are no muscles in the lungs themselves to make them fill up or empty out. Some of the action comes from the muscles of the ribs and chest. The whole rib cage expands and contracts and that helps move the air. But the secret to deep breathing isn't the chest; it's the diaphragm.

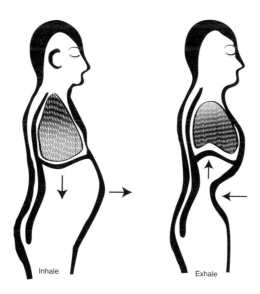

Lungs and diaphragm: inhale and exhale, sitting up.

The diaphragm is a broad sheet of muscle underneath the lungs. It's like a thick tarp, separating what's above it—the heart and lungs—from what's below—the stomach and digestive track, liver, kidneys, bladder, and pancreas.

Sit up straight. Push out your stomach as if you're trying to look pregnant or as if you have a beer belly. As you push your belly outward, the diaphragm drops down because the intestines underneath have been partially displaced.

Now pull in your stomach. This will bring the partially displaced intestines back under the diaphragm, which will push it upward.

Repeat this a few times until you can make the motion easily. Don't bother inhaling and exhaling yet; just practice pushing the stomach out and then pulling it back in.

Master the Motion

If you're having difficulty isolating the abdominal muscles, try to do it lying on your back with a small weight (like a book) on your belly. As you inhale, make the book rise using just the force of your lower abdominal muscles. As you exhale, contract the stomach muscles and let the book lower down. Do this smoothly, with no jerking or quick moves. This will force you to use the stomach muscles to accomplish the movement, instead of cheating by using your back or shoulder muscles.

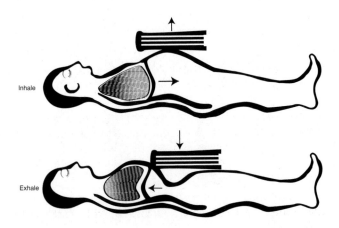

Lungs and diaphragm: inhale and exhale lying down, with weight.

Now sit up and try it again in front of the mirror. When you get the stomach motion easily, watch your chest and shoulders, too, and make sure they aren't moving. Let all the work happen from the lower abdomen. Your center of gravity is about 3 inches below the belly button and back a bit, about halfway between your belly button and your spine. That's where the push forward and the contraction back should come from. The mirror can be your low-tech biofeedback machine for learning these skills.

It might sound complicated at first, but the breath I'm describing is actually a natural process. If you watch a sleeping baby breathe, she's doing exactly what I'm describing. The funny thing is that if I had started this chapter by asking you to take the deepest breath you could, almost all beginners would have done the exact opposite: your chest and shoulders would have risen, you would have tried to expand your rib cage, and you probably would have sniffed the breath upward instead of back and down into the throat. Now why is that?

My theory is the popularization of the famous army command, "Stomach in; chest out." How many physical education teachers have you heard using that one? It's great for looking good in your uniform or standing in line; it's horrible when you're trying to take a really deep breath. Using that command, I can breathe in for four or five seconds at most. Doing the opposite—belly out; belly in—I can inhale for over 20 seconds.

Now add the breath to your belly movements. Inhale as you push the belly out, lowering the diaphragm and allowing the lungs to fill the empty space. Try to inhale slowly, counting 1-2-3-4 seconds in your mind. Don't raise your shoulders and don't move your chest. Do all the work from the abdomen. When you feel your lungs are full, reverse the breath and exhale as you contract your abdominal muscles.

stay Grounded

Always keep your eyes open during any of the breathing exercises in this book. And, for now, only practice them sitting down. If you get lightheaded at all, stop all practice, keep your eyes open, and wait until the feeling passes. Then don't do anything for a few more minutes. After that, you can slowly try it again.

As you inhale, remember to breathe back and down toward the throat, not upward into the nasal cavity.

Before you move on to the breathing exercises, I recommend you spend some time with these instructions. Read them through a few times to be certain that you're doing exactly what I'm describing and doing. And if you have any health concerns about undertaking a basic breathing routine, consult your physician before you begin.

There's one more thing to learn before you get to the individual exercises. You may need the mirror for this one because it's tricky, and if you do it incorrectly, you can lose the abdominal control you've developed so far.

Think of the two steps you've followed so far.

1. Inhale slowly through the nose (back and down into the back of the throat) while simultaneously pushing your lower belly out.

2. Exhale slowly, through the mouth, as if you're whispering the word "hah" as you contract the belly in.

Now, pretend those aren't steps one and two, but rather steps one and four. They're the steps for inhaling and exhaling. Now we're going to add two quick middle motions, steps two and three.

2. With your belly out (and your lungs full), inhale a little more as you lift your pushed-out belly just a bit. It's as if you're swinging your bellybutton back in and up a bit while simultaneously taking in a little more air. And do it without raising your chest or shoulders.

3. Exhale a little bit, the same amount of air you took in, in step 2. Take the first count of the exhalation and put the stomach back where it was in step 1. As you exhale with "hah," push the stomach back down and out.

So the sequence of the four steps is now:

1. Inhale in the nose, back and down into the throat, as you push the belly out.

2. Inhale in the nose, swinging the bellybutton in and up slightly, allowing the front of the diaphragm to come forward without moving the chest or shoulders.

3. Exhale out of the mouth, whispering "hah," as you drop the belly down and out again, back to its first position.

4. Continue to exhale out of the mouth, continuing to whisper "hah," as you forcibly pull the belly back in.

To simplify even further, the belly movements are as follows:

1. Belly out

2. Belly up

3. Belly down

4. Belly in

The four breath steps, simultaneous to the belly moves, are these:

1. Inhale

2. Inhale

3. Exhale

4. Exhale

Once you've mastered these four steps, the three breaths described next will be a piece of cake. The main differences between them are in the timing. Use the videos listed in the Resources appendix to help you along.

The Cleansing Breath

The cleansing breath is a great way to start any breathing session. It cleans the lungs and wakes up the diaphragm to let it know there's some serious breath-work ahead.

1. Inhale as deeply as possible, allowing the stomach to expand forward as you do. Do this slowly, divided over three seconds.

2. Continue to inhale. At the very end of the inhalation, during the last second (the fourth count), bring the stomach up.

3. Before you exhale, without any breath, drop the belly back to the first position.

4. Relax the throat and exhale forcibly, contracting the abdominal muscles inward as sharply and quickly as you can.

To help amplify the power necessary for the cleansing breath, try this: As you go through steps 1 through 3, bring your hands up and back to your ribs, palms out and fingers pointing up, in a surrendering kind of position, but at the ribcage height. Then, on step 4, as you exhale, push your hands forward sharply, away from your ribs—palms open, fingers pointing upward—as if you were shoving a piano on wheels across the room.

Repeat three times.

The next two breaths are the even breath and the pacing breath. I've chosen them for a very specific reason.

The average person breathes about 15 breaths per minute (bpm) in a waking state. That means that each breath is about four seconds, so inhale for two seconds and exhale for two seconds.

If we were to speed up our breath to 30 bpm or slow it down to 7.5 bpm, we might send a signal to the autonomic nervous system that we were in a sympathetic (fight-or-flight) or parasympathetic (relaxation) zone, which would enable us to charge ourselves up or relax. Either way, the rate of the breath, above or below your normal sitting rate, is what initiates the change. These are exercises for the autonomic nervous system and, practiced together, will help balance the energy matrix.

In Dr. Puharich's seminal work *Beyond Telepathy*, he explained how yogis and shamans—and Sufism's "whirling dervishes" and Hasidic dancers as well—all had practices that began with very fast movements that stimulated faster breathing, followed by moments of silence afterward, which initiated slower breathing. He observed that the stronger the adrenergic (sympathetic) response caused by the faster movement and breath, the deeper the cholinergic (parasympathetic) response afterward. In other words, the higher you jump on the diving board, the deeper you go into the water. Because the goal was to have a charged-up energy matrix with a deep-trance state, they began with the faster, stronger movement and breath. That's why I'm giving you the steps for the faster pacing breath first and the slower, even breath immediately after it. Always practice them together.

The Pacing Breath

This is called the pacing breath because it's excellent to use while walking vigorously or doing aerobic exercises. It will help you generate and control the extra oxygen and energy you'll need. It is simply mirroring what your system does by causing faster breathing for faster energy demands.

stay
Grounded

The pacing breath, when used as part of the breathing series in this chapter, must be practiced with eyes open and sitting down because the breath might cause some lightheadedness. If you follow it immediately with the slow, even breath, that feeling will disappear very quickly.

1. Inhale quickly and vigorously, in a quick, half-second count. Be sure to inhale through the nose, back and down into the throat, as you push the belly goes out.

2. Inhale quickly, in another half-second count, swinging the bellybutton in and up slightly, allowing the front of the diaphragm to come forward. Don't move your chest or shoulders.

3. Exhale, quickly and vigorously, in a quick, half-second count, out the mouth while whispering "hah," as you drop the belly down and out again, back to where you were at the end of the first step.

4. Continue to exhale, quickly and vigorously, in a final half-second count, out the mouth while continuing to whisper "hah," as you forcibly pull the belly back in.

As you practice this breath, imagine that it's a very hot day and you're rapidly splashing invigorating cold water on yourself to cool off. It's intended to charge you up, and your imagination is an important element.

Repeat this breath 15 to 30 times for best effect. It takes two seconds for the complete pacing breath sequence, meaning that if you do it properly, you should be doubling your average breath rate of 15 bpm to 30 bpm. It will charge your system with increased energy and gently speed up your pulse and heart rate. The videos referred to in the resource section of Appendix B (see www.andronenergyhealing.org) will help make this very clear.

In time, you can gradually increase the timing and repetitions to 60 breaths per minute. Be sure, when you attempt that increase, that you don't lose the vigorous nature of the breath.

The Even Breath

Finally, we come to the breath you'll probably use more than any other. It's called the even breath for two reasons. The first is obvious: the inhalation and exhalation are even—four counts each. The second is that it will slow you down and even you out in stressful times. You'll be lowering your bpm to 7.5, which is half the normal rate.

1. Inhale for three seconds, in the nose, back and down into the throat, and as you push the belly goes out.

2. Inhale for one more second, in the nose, swinging the bellybutton in and up slightly, allowing the front of the diaphragm to come forward. Don't move your chest or shoulders.

3. Exhale for one second, out the mouth while whispering "hah," as you drop the belly down and out again, back to the ending position of the first step.

4. Continue to exhale for three more seconds, out the mouth while continuing to whisper "hah," as you forcibly pull the belly back in.

Unlike the pacing breath, which is intended to stimulate and invigorate, the even breath is designed to quiet you down. When practicing it, visualize the calm, even flow of relaxing energy filling your body as tension and stress are eliminated.

In time, this breath will become second nature to you. It's possible to increase the breath to a deeper practice by increasing the duration of each inhalation one count at a time—a 5:5, 6:6, 7:7, or 8:8 count. If you choose to do this, keep three things in mind:

1. Perform each count without any stress or strain before you move to a slower count.

2. Always maintain the 1:1 ratio as you increase the numbers. It's 4:4, not 4:5 or 4:6.

3. Never change the duration of steps 2 and 3. They're *always* one count. The increase will be done on the first and fourth steps: 4-1:1-4 or 5-1:1-5 and so forth.

If you find yourself filling up too quickly, focus on really pushing that belly out on the first count. And push it out from as low behind the bellybutton as you can. When you're breathing properly from that low point, the center of gravity, you'll find it much easier to increase the duration of the inhalation.

Deeper connections
People with yoga experience will ask why I'm not teaching the popular 1:2 ratio (inhale 4, exhale 8). The 4:8 breath is also designed for deep relaxation, but in my opinion it isn't the best set to start with. It doesn't give you enough time to really master the individual steps. In time, that becomes easy, too.

There are a great number of breaths and ratios of breaths I haven't even touched on: the bellows breath, for example, is practiced in birthing classes all over the world. There are breaths to speed up the body, slow down the body, cool the body, warm the body, and even breaths to massage and relax the vocal cords. I'm familiar with more than 75 different breaths and practice at least 25 of them regularly, but I've found these three breaths provide the perfect foundation for breath-work.

Homework

Here's a basic homework guide for beginning breath-work. This whole set can be done in three minutes or less once you've mastered the breaths. Don't try to extend breath duration until you can do this set easily and comfortably.

Suggested Breath Series for Beginners

3–5 Cleansing Breaths	Inhale 4 : Exhale 1
15–30 Pacing Breaths	Inhale 1 : Exhale 1
7–10 Even Breaths	Inhale 4 : Exhale 4

Essential Takeaways

- Breath-work is a universally utilized method of quieting the mind and energizing the body and energy matrix.

- Different breathing techniques have different effects on the system: energizing, calming, warmth, focus, etc.

- Breathing faster energizes the system, and breathing more slowly relaxes it; the two breaths should be practiced together for maximum energy balance and effectiveness in energy healing, and to exercise the autonomic nervous system.

- Until you've mastered control of the abdominal muscles and diaphragm, practice breath-work with a mirror.

- Follow the rules about posture and the position of eyes, nose, and throat; they'll greatly enhance your breath-work.

chapter 14

Rooting: Doing Energy Work Safely

Grounding yourself for energy centering

Exercises for finding your center

The five steps of rooting

Practical applications in everyday life

The idea of centering oneself—finding a state of equilibrium in mind, body, and spirit—is found in every system of personal growth and spiritual development. Centering has even found its way into the more mainstream vocabulary as a tool for stress management.

Centering is about finding your real center so that when a challenging moment of force attacks or confronts you, you're able to yield rather than fall victim to it. By knowing who you are on the deepest level possible, you know that you're doing your best at what you believe to be your purpose in life. When looked at from that perspective, criticism doesn't hurt; it shows you where you can improve. And praise doesn't necessarily inflate you; it can show you how far you've come, but also how far you have left to go.

There's a good test of this principle in the martial arts. In traditional systems, when you're practicing free-style combat and are struck by your opponent, you're taught to say "thank you." Your opponent has just taught you where your defenses were weak by striking you there. He deserves your thanks, not your anger. It's a good test of where that ego is; "What? Thank him for hitting me? Are you crazy?" is not the response we're looking for.

There are dozens, if not hundreds, of techniques out there to help you find your center. We're going to focus on one called rooting.

The Rooting Process

Rooting, based on a martial arts technique, has specific applications and usefulness for energy healing. Variations of this technique or principle (under different names such as grounding or centering) are found in many energy healing systems. The idea is that you find your physical center of gravity and learn how to attach your body's center with the earth, to become immovable. An attacker may try to push you over or break a hold you've got him in, but he can't. You're rooted to the earth like a tree.

Two systems of martial arts are well known for rooting: *Aikido* and t'ai chi ch'uan.

Finding Meaning

Aikido, known for using the force of the attacker to defeat him by redirecting that force from a centered state, is relatively new in the martial arts world. Grand Master Morihei Uyeshiba developed it in the early twentieth century. The Japanese word means *the way* (dō, or Tao) *of unifying (or sinking Ai) the life energy* (ki, or qi).

If you've ever tried to pull a puppy or a young child somewhere when she doesn't want to go, you've experienced the phenomenon of rooting. They instinctively lower their centers of gravity and manifest greater strength than you'd expect.

I've offered dramatic demonstrations of rooting on stage when I've asked a very strong person in the audience to come up and lift my wife. Lillian, at 4'10" and under 100 pounds, allows herself to be lifted by the volunteer, who might be a professional football player or a weightlifter who could easily bench 400 pounds. Then she roots, and to the amazement of the audience and the total disbelief of the weightlifter, she's unmovable. Without changing her physical position she's able to simply change her mind as to whether they can lift her or not. When Lillian first began, it would take her a few moments to get herself into that state. Now, an experienced third-degree black belt with almost 40 years' experience, she does it in an instant.

When Dr. Puharich, the scientist with whom I spent so much time, saw this demonstration, he immediately began to contemplate the science behind it. He had a hypothesis that rooting was related to an "increase in the gravitational constant by an act of will in the positive polarization of quarks and magnetic monopoles," whatever that means, but we never had the opportunity to test it any further.

For our purposes in energy healing, rooting is a psychophysical technique for getting in touch with, and learning to control, the vast living energies in and around us. Not to sound like a broken record, but we live in a WEB, an ocean of energy, all the time. Our purpose is to try to attune ourselves to an awareness of this energy.

There are two important applications of the rooting process in energy healing. First, the roots that grab the center of the earth are obviously not physical; they're made of energy. Imagining energy roots connecting to the center of the earth is the same as having your energy matrix phase-lock with the beat of the earth. When you're rooted, you're able to access energy from the earth to upgrade your energy matrix to increase your energy potential.

The roots can also work in reverse, grounding us against harmful energy and redirecting it away from us. A direct hit from a lightning bolt can destroy a house, but if you put a lightning rod at the highest point of the house, the rod will attract the electric surge. It will then redirect that harmful electricity down a wire into the earth, bypassing the house.

We've already discussed the idea that words have real energy. If a harmful word-attack comes at you and you're rooted—meaning that your center is connected to the earth's center—the energy of that attack will pass right through you, leaving you unaffected, just as the house was unaffected by the lightning bolt.

In Chapter 4, we utilized a muscle-testing and saw how the muscle went weak when we sent a verbal stressor at the subject. We don't even have to say it aloud; just thinking negative thoughts can weaken the muscle.

However, if we did the same test on a rooted subject we'd see that when the subject is rooted, the verbal or thought attack is nullified and the arm stays strong. The roots serve as our lightning rod.

Imagine you're a teacher and you've just announced a pop quiz. At that moment, you know your 25 students are sending some less-than-wonderful thoughts in your direction. Will the energy of those negative thoughts affect your meridians and weaken your muscles? They will—but because you know it's coming, you can do something about it. You can root, activating an internal energy lightning rod and grounding the energy attack.

As magical as this sounds, it does work. When looked at from an energy perspective, our thoughts—and everyone else's—are energy, and as such, have an influence on everything around us. If someone else sends a negative thought your way, it can have a hurtful effect on your energy matrix. In the case of our muscle test exercise, it weakens the energy flow through our arm, making the arm go weak. By rooting, you are boosting the power to your energy matrix, grounding you against these hurtful energy attacks. If you're able to do this successfully during the muscle test, your arm will remain strong.

Games to Find Your Center of Gravity

Before we go into the step-by-step aspect of meditative rooting, let's start with some games we often play in martial arts classes to help find our physical centers. From there it's a smaller leap to the concept of an energy center or a mental and emotional center. You'll need a partner to practice these games.

Centering Game 1: Stand with your feet about a foot apart. Relax and bend your knees. Now have someone stand in front of you and put her right hand on your left shoulder, or vice verse, and push firmly but smoothly.

Chances are you stumbled backward. Now try again, but this time focus on your center (below the navel) and imagine yourself being tied by an unbreakable cable to the center of the earth. Relax your shoulders and yield to the pressure of the push. Your shoulder should give way as your body rotates (from your center) and remains standing.

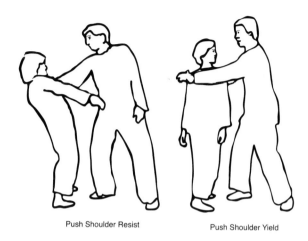

Push Shoulder Resist   Push Shoulder Yield

Centering game #1.

Centering Game 2: Stand opposite your opponent at arm's length, both with your feet about a foot apart. Put your hands at chest height, palms facing your opponent. Try to slap each other's hands hard enough to knock the other person back.

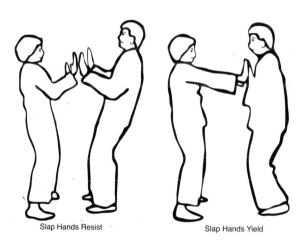

Slap Hands Resist   Slap Hands Yield

Centering game #2.

The winner is the one who doesn't fall backward, losing his balance. You'll learn very quickly that when you're slapped, you must yield. The key is to hit the other player's hands when that person has muscular tension in the arms and shoulders; that is, when she doesn't yield. With a little practice you'll learn to relax your upper torso and shift your weight to the natural center of gravity below the navel.

These games are an excellent way to zero in on your physical center to root more effectively.

As you practice these games, make sure you have enough room on all sides. Until you get good at working from your center of gravity, you may fall backward or to the side, and you don't want to break your grandmother's antique lamp when you do.

As you know, I like to focus first on the attitude needed to facilitate the practice of a new skill. Years ago, I wrote this little verse for my first black belt students. It's a compilation of many of the wonderful lessons my teachers taught me about "being like a tree," which is what you're imagining as you prepare to root.

> *BE LIKE A TREE*
>
> *Balanced, centered, understanding nature's plan*
>
> *BE LIKE A TREE*
>
> *Flexible, bending to the storms of change without breaking*
>
> *BE LIKE A TREE*
>
> *An individual, yet tuned to the vibrations of the whole*
>
> *BE LIKE A TREE*
>
> *Moderate in your demands and expectations*
>
> *BE LIKE A TREE*
>
> *Rooted for survival, reaching upward toward the light,*
>
> *and bearing your fruits in season*

The key element, of course, is that when we see ourselves as part of the whole and not the center of everything, we can handle the stressors and transitions that are always around us without being blown over. This is the Yield part of Y.E.S., the preparatory attitude that precedes effective Energizing.

The Technique of Rooting

The rooting process is very simple. Begin to breathe at a rate of 4:4, with the even breath you learned in Chapter 13. Do that for at least a minute (about 7 breaths) or until you feel relaxed and quiet. Let go of the muscular tension in your face and hands. Keep your neck and shoulders free of tension. Allow your eyes to close if you'd like; most people do, once they've learned the technique. As you inhale and exhale, imagine that your breaths are the waves at the beach, coming up to the shore and going back out to sea. Clear your mind of random thoughts. Imagine that your thoughts are like footprints in the sand and the waves of your breathing can just wash them away.

Now we're ready to proceed to the five steps of the rooting process: open, silence, center, attune, root (or O.S.C.A.R.).

Open

Open your mind to the idea that you, and all the earth, are living vibrations and that you can feel that vibration and make it your own. Imagine you just beamed in from the *Enterprise* and you haven't become solid yet. You're an energy matrix, sitting on top of a planet that's pure energy, inside the WEB.

Open your inner eye. Now, as your physical eyes close, open an imaginary eye at the base of your skull, on the back of your head. Imagine that with that eye of imagination, you can sense the energy world around you; you can see-hear-feel with it.

Silence

Be still … be passive … be ready. Listen carefully to the sound of your breath as it flows inside your head; feel its vibration. Now, use your imaginary eye, the one at the back of your head, to look forward, inside your head. Imagine a seed of light floating inside, at the center of your head. Imagine it floating like a speck of dust on a sunbeam coming in your window on a warm afternoon. Imagine that seed of light filling your head with a silent light. It's gentle and still. We'll call this place inside your head, where the seed rests, the upper center.

Rooting

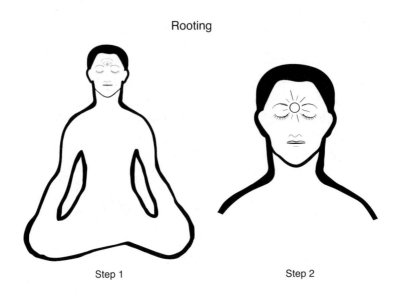

Step 1   Step 2

Rooting step 1: open.

Rooting step 2: silence.

Center

Now imagine the seed of light floating down from the upper center in your head—slowly, like a pearl sinking downward in a jar of honey—to the lower center of your body, about 3 inches below and behind your navel. As it floats down, imagine that the seed of light is leaving a trail of light in its wake, a trail of silence. Everything the seed touches becomes still, becomes tranquil. The seed comes to rest at your lower center, directly behind the abdominal muscles you're using in your slow 4-4 even breath.

Attune

Attune your energy matrix to the silent vibration of the seed at the lower center. With each breath, imagine the seed growing brighter and brighter, as if you're turning a dimmer up with every breath you take. Imagine its light radiating outward, lighting up the whole energy matrix. As it reaches each part of your energy body, it attunes the energy matrix to the silent heartbeat of the seed. It rises up to your head and goes beyond its physical shell, attuning whatever it lights upon. It goes down your legs and beyond them; it fills your torso and goes out to your arms and beyond your fingertips. Imagine the entire energy matrix attuned to that frequency of healing silence. Imagine your beautiful, glowing energy matrix, attuned to the vibration of the seed and of the 8 hz heartbeat of the earth itself. The seed is ready to sprout.

Rooting

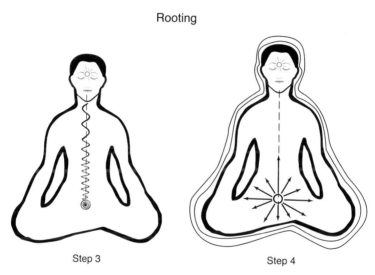

Step 3   Step 4

Rooting step 3: center. Rooting step 4: attune.

Root

As the seed sprouts, imagine two laser-like roots of light sinking from the lower center within your energy matrix—where the seed is—to a pool of light at the center of the earth. Imagine those roots connecting your energy matrix's lower center to the earth center, in an inseparable bond, becoming one.

When that image is perfectly clear in your mind's eye, your energy matrix's upper center joined to the earth center, with those laser-like roots of light, gently bring your first three fingers together on each hand and touch the tips together and hold them there. Try to focus on three things simultaneously: feel the fingers touching, hear the word "root" silently in your head, and imagine that image of your energy matrix rooted to the earth. Keep your thumb touching the tips of the index and middle fingers, and hold them softly together. You are rooted.

Rooting

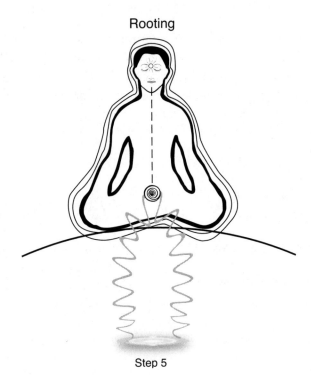

Step 5

Rooting step 5: root.

Deeper connections

Touching the fingers together provides a tactile anchor to help you root more quickly the next time you do it. It's what hypnotherapists used to call a post-hypnotic suggestion but today call an anchor. Do it together with hearing the word root and seeing the image of the roots. The anchor will be multisensory and the rooting will be deepened.

Qi Gung and Rooting Energy Exercises

Now that you're rooted, let's do a couple of exercises to use your roots.

Energy Filtering

Let's use your roots to clean out some of the plaque (tension, stress, anxiety, fear, pain, disease, etc.) from your energy matrix. As you exhale, imagine any energy plaque going down the roots and entering the pool of light at the center of the planet. Imagine it being cleansed in the pool of light. Now, as you inhale, imagine that filtered energy coming back up into your energy matrix, refreshed, recycled, and revitalized. Continue this in a series of 7–10 breaths; I think you'll find it very refreshing.

Energy Biofeedback

I promised earlier that I'd help you install an internal biofeedback machine—and here it is.

First, go through the five steps of rooting: open, silence, center, attune, and root (O.S.C.A.R.). Continue to breathe evenly with your hands palm up on your lap, your fingers touching in the rooted position. Now let your inner eye of imagination gaze down from within you to the pool of light at the center of the planet. Slowly release the fingertips and rotate your hands so they're palms down, resting on the tops of your thighs. Hold on to the feeling of being rooted and connected to the pool of light.

Now, as you inhale slowly (4:4), raise your arms upward to about shoulder height, imagining that you're drawing energy up the roots, from the pool of light, into your energy matrix. There should be no tension at all in your shoulders or fingers. As you exhale, let your hands float down to just above, but not touching, your legs. Keep your hands light, as if they're floating on a cloud. Repeat this three times, each inhalation timed with the raising of your arms and each exhalation timed with the lowering of your arms.

After the third cycle, bring your hands up and turn them inward, as if you're holding a basketball of energy in front of you. Be very gentle with that ball, as if it's a bubble about to pop. Slowly stretch it out about an inch in each direction, then come to a stop and press it back in just a hair.

Repeat that three times: out an inch, back just a hair; out an inch, back just a hair. Naturally your hands are a few inches farther apart now, as each motion took you outward just a bit.

Now try this: Leaving your left hand where it is, draw only your right hand out a bit. Then, as you bring the right hand back in, imagine that the energy bubble in your right hand is pushing the left hand. Slowly bring the right hand to a stop as the left hand moves out and, as the left hand moves back in, the energy bubble pushes the right hand again. Go back and forth a few times, from right to left, trying to feel the energy of the bubble between your hands.

If you feel any sensation, you're doing it right. It might feel as if two magnets are pushing each other with their magnetic fields, or you may feel a gentle heat or coolness. Others feel a breeze between the two.

This is your energy biofeedback machine. When you feel that sensation of energy between your hands, you'll know you're rooted, and that your energy matrix is phase-locked with the 8 hz heartbeat of the earth.

This exercise is a basic way to get in touch with your energy matrix. If you feel this energy in your hands naturally, great! But I cannot encourage you enough to go through the steps of rooting (or some other similar system you may practice that does the same thing) before you begin energy healing. To work with energy safely, you must be grounded. After a while it may only take a single thought to do that.

Back to Basics

MISC.

Even when an idea comes naturally to you, practice is always recommended. Vladimir Horowortz, the piano virtuoso, widely considered one of the greatest piano players of the twentieth century, would often practice musical scales on the fold-down trays on airplanes! You can never have too much mastery over the basics.

For Best Results

To become a true master of rooting could take a lifetime. Here are a few tips and tricks to help get those roots moving a little more quickly.

Repetition

Remember, practice makes permanent. For best results, practice each step in the O.S.C.A.R. sequence for 3–5 breaths (the 4:4 even breaths). The entire sequence should take approximately three minutes. Try to do it 3–5 times a day for a month. By the end of that time, you should be quite proficient at rooting.

It's always a good time to root, but the best moments during the day are first thing in the morning and right before bed. It's also a good idea to root before stressful events like performances or presentations, or before exams or interviews.

For me, one of the best times to practice is just before meals. The advantage is that I become relaxed before I begin to eat, so my food is digested more thoroughly. Practicing before meals can be especially helpful for people who eat on the run.

Imagination

As strange as it may sound, it helps to have a good imagination. That's not to say that rooting is imaginary; far from it. Energy is real, but the more clearly you can visualize or imagine it, the more effective your rooting will be.

For years I imagined these roots when I engaged in energy healing and taught them many thousands of times. One afternoon Dr. Puharich called and said he was driving past my home with someone he wanted me to meet. He told me that she—let's call her SA—was one of the most powerful psychics he'd ever worked with. She was able to look inside the atom and describe what she saw and to look inside the body to diagnose it.

When they arrived, Dr. Puharich asked if I would do some energy healing on him; he'd been having some health problems. SA described what my aura was doing as I worked, and her accuracy was uncanny. She was able to see and describe everything I was doing, without being told, 10 out of 10 times. When I focused on his liver, she said something was going on with the liver and she could see it!

But it was actually the first thing she said that blew my mind. As I rooted and began to work, she said, "I'm seeing energy lines coming from your lower abdomen and going down into the earth; do you know what that could be?" We'd never met; she knew nothing about me, or about rooting, but she was able to see something that I'd only imagined.

Just because you imagine something doesn't mean it isn't real.

Mind Over Energy Over Matter

Raise your arm straight up and then lower it. Okay; how did you do it? And don't tell me about neurons and synapses and bones and muscles, because you didn't give them a second's thought. You raised your hand by imagining it going upward and it did. You were able to create a picture, an image, in your mind and supply it with some will power and some energy to make it happen. If you can raise your arm with your mind, you can certainly move energy with your mind; it has far less resistance.

I've seen imagination be the difference between success and failure in energy work. In 1979, Lillian was training to receive her black belt. Because of her size, she was concerned about the breaking requirement; she would have to break 5 inches of wood or stone with her hand in order to pass. It wasn't going to be done with any kind of brute force, that's for sure. She was going to need to tap into a greater energy to accomplish it (which is actually the whole point of the requirement).

During a class one day, she set up the boards and struck them repeatedly with no success. Her physical technique was excellent, but the boards wouldn't break. I told her she really had to focus.

> "Imagine you're an energy being. You're drawing energy up from the center of the earth. Imagine it's going into your arm and then imagine a laser pulse of concentrated light cutting through those boards, just as lasers cut through steel."

She vehemently demanded,

> "Are you telling me that after six years of trying to master stances, breathing, action/reaction in

movement, focus, and technique, that the difference between being a brown belt and a black belt is *imagination*?"

"Yes! That's exactly what I'm telling you!"

Well, she imagined. The boards broke, and the rest is history. She was awarded the first woman's black belt in our style's history.

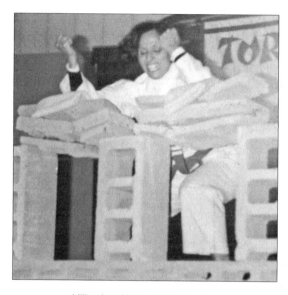

Lillian breaking concrete blocks.

Know Thyself

There are a lot of different kinds of learners and thinkers. To succeed with the rooting process, it helps to know what kind of thinker you are to best focus your training.

If you're a visual person, imagine seeing your body made of energy. If you're more of an aural person, hearing the words open, silence, center, attune, and root as you go through the steps may be more useful than trying to imagine pictures. For the kinesthetic, the touching of the thumb to the first two fingers may be the most important step.

Of course, the very best way is to do all three: imagine that you see the roots, feel your fingers touch, and hear the word root inside your head as you say it to yourself. Remember, we're all a combination of visual, aural, and kinesthetic anyway.

The Instant Root

There are times when stress needs to be grounded instantly, and you won't have time to do a full 3-to-5-minute meditation. Remember that teacher announcing a surprise quiz to her class? She'll be at the receiving end of 25 negative energy attacks within seconds! What should she do? There's a simple technique for those emergencies.

When you need to root, and fast, use the rooting anchor we established earlier. Make a circle in the air with your thumb, forefinger, and middle finger, so the fingers are about 2 or 3 inches apart. As you draw your fingers together, imagine that they're closing an electrical circuit, allowing energy to flow up into your body. Feel the energy circulating all through your body and then flowing back into the earth. This circuit of energy will ground the stressor energy, dissipate it, and revitalize your energy matrix with healthy energy.

Deeper Connections

A great time for the instant root is during a business meeting. Stressful situations call for being grounded, but if you close your eyes and start meditating in the board room, you're likely to be committed! No one will notice if you do the instant root with your fingers under the table, and you'll be more effective in the meeting.

It may take some practice to get this technique to work for you, but if you use it every day when you practice your regular rooting exercises, it will eventually become an automatic signal to your energy matrix to activate the rooting process. The longer you hold your fingers together, the longer the energy flow will continue. When you let go, the energy flow will return to its normal pace.

The instant root is fine for occasional use, but when you have the time, use the longer routine.

Uses of Rooting

There are many practical uses for the rooting process. Use it to …

- Ground stress by making your body a lightning rod that allows threatening and stressful energy to pass through without harming your body or your energy matrix.

- Get to sleep by extending the rooting energy out to your fingers and toes.

- Heal yourself by mentally draining away negative, sick energy and drawing in positive, healthy energy.

- Achieve a quiet mental state that will free up your creativity and problem-solving abilities. This will enable you to reprogram your mental computer so you can radiate an effective presence in personal and business encounters.

Most importantly, rooting provides the philosophical basis for dealing with stress. It's of fundamental importance that values such as responsibility, patience, perseverance, humility, and moderation in all things—the values offered to us by the great philosophies and religions—become realities in our daily lives. It's not enough for us to talk about these values; we have to put them into practice, for our own personal evolution as well as the evolution of our planet. With that in mind, the rooting process takes on great meaning and relevance for our lives and our world.

Remember, the strength of a tree lies in its ability to root deep into the ground. So be like a tree. That's the essence of rooting.

Essential Takeaways

- Rooting is a centering technique for getting you in touch with your energy matrix and logging on to the WEB.
- By rooting, you can draw positive energy up from the center of the earth and also ground yourself quickly against harmful energy.
- Give yourself an O.S.C.A.R.: open, silence, center, attune, root.
- Be patient and perseverant. The more you practice it correctly, the better you get.

chapter 15

Ocular Divergence to Facilitate Energy Healing

One of nature's unsung methods to relax the mind

Basic exercises for ocular divergence

Uncoupling the hemispheres with eyes, ears, and nose

A simple technique called ocular divergence can help you relax quickly, assist your getting into an alpha state, and help your energy matrix log on to the WEB, the earth's energy. It's been used for millennia in a variety of ways to achieve the same results. It can improve learning and test scores in school, as well as your effectiveness in energy healing. But while most of us do it every day without even realizing it, very few people know about it, so they haven't learned how to do it better. This chapter will remedy that situation. I'll also discuss two other forms of divergence to amplify your progress.

What Is Ocular Divergence?

In Chapter 3, I mentioned briefly that ocular divergence is one of the best ways to achieve an alpha 8 hz brain rhythm. Let's see how we normally see things so we can understand how ocular divergence is different.

The Theory Behind It

When we look at something, each eye sees a flat, 2-dimensional image and sends that image to the brain. Because the eyes are a few inches apart, they each see the image from a slightly different angle. You can test that by looking at an object with one eye covered and then switching to the other eye. The object seems to be moving back and forth. Obviously it's not; the apparent movement is caused by the fact that you're seeing the object from two different points of view. Literally!

If you keep both eyes open the object changes again. Now it appears 3-dimensional. The brain has taken the two images you sent it and put them together to create a third way of looking at the object. That's exactly how the View-Master® toys work: Two pictures are taken of a scene from slightly different points of view, simulating the way your eyes each see it, and put on two slides. When you look at the images with *both* eyes, it appears in 3-D.

Check This Out

MISC.

Hold a pencil vertically about a foot away from your eyes. Close one eye and look at it. Then switch eyes. The object appears to move. Go back and forth a few times and notice the change. Finally, open both eyes and pay careful attention to how the third image is 3-dimensional, not flat like the other two.

To understand ocular divergence, imagine that each of your eyes has a red laser connecting it to the object you're looking at; a pencil, for instance. The angle formed by the two lasers looks like a triangle because the lasers start at the eyes (a few inches apart) and meet at the pencil (a single point). Depending on how far away the object is, the angle of the lines will change; an object closer to you will have a larger degree than the object farther away, but in the end they always meet, or converge.

What would happen if you could make the two lines become almost parallel to each other, so that they never touched at all? The lines don't converge at the object you're looking at; they diverge.

Here's why the difference is so important: each of your eyes is linked to one of the hemispheres of your brain. The left eye is linked to the right hemisphere and the right eye is linked to the left. While both hemispheres are busy all day battling for supremacy, both eyes are busy feeding information to the brain. When you achieve ocular divergence, the two hemispheres uncouple, giving both eyes and the brain a rest. It's like sending a message to the brain to uncouple and relax.

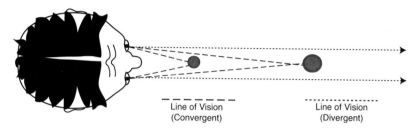

Line of Vision
(Convergent)

Line of Vision
(Divergent)

Eyes in Convergence

Lines of vision in convergence and divergence.

I've seen this demonstrated in Dr. Puharich's lab and had it performed on myself. Brain wave measurements can be taken of the individual hemispheres independently. When the eyes diverge, the brain wave consistently slows down, bringing you to a relaxed alpha state faster.

You can see it for yourself without any fancy equipment. Looking into a mirror, watch how the pupils of your eyes dilate as you enter the divergent state. The pupils normally dilate and contract to balance the amount of light that enters your eyes, but if there's no change in light, they won't change on their own. Think of a modern camera; the aperture opens and closes automatically. But a photographer can manually adjust the aperture for a particular effect, and that's what you're doing when you practice ocular divergence. You're basically overriding the default settings on your eyes. The pupils dilate as you uncouple the hemispheres and enter a light trance state.

Peripheral Vision, Learning, and Stress

Simply stated, ocular divergence is when your eyes, which normally focus to the same point in front of you, each focus straight ahead instead. Your field of vision—what you see in front of you and *peripherally*—expands.

Your **peripheral field of vision (FOV)** is determined by how wide an angle you can see to the farthest points on your right and left. Try this: Close your right eye and place your left finger as far out to the left as possible until you can't see it anymore. Then do the same with your right finger. The angle formed by both fingers, relative to your eye, is your FOV for that eye. Now try it with the other eye.

A fascinating book, *Light: Medicine of the Future,* by Dr. Jacob Liberman, DO, PhD, analyzes how the more stress we're under, the smaller our field of vision becomes. And that's made even worse if we're out of balance in diet, rest, or ability to cope.

Using what he called syntonic therapy, he found that in 20-minute sessions, 4 times a week for 6 weeks, he was able to expand the field of vision, which had a dramatic effect on a number of problems, including hyperactivity in children. He reported that with this therapy, many children calmed down, there was a 75 percent improvement in schoolwork and a 40 percent improvement in handwriting, and kids who had been withdrawn became more outgoing.

While I haven't conducted any controlled laboratory experiments with the techniques in ocular divergence you're about to learn, I've seen tremendous improvement in hundreds of students over the years in managing stress, as well as specific cases that showed improvement in learning, diet, and allergies, all connected to the combination of breathing, rooting, and ocular divergence training.

I was first exposed to ocular divergence skills as part of my martial arts training. We focused on expanding peripheral vision to sense oncoming attacks without losing an inner sense of calm and centeredness. That kind of training has been around for centuries. Hypnosis teaches that when we are in a light trance, our pupils dilate. It's all connected.

Revealing the Third Triasphere

If the hemispheres are uncoupled, and thereby somewhat at rest, it begs the question: which part of the mind is receiving information?

According to Kabbalistic theory, there are three levels of knowledge: Ḥoch'mah, Binah, and Da'at. Think of the right brain as the receiver for Ḥoch'mah (intuitive wisdom) and the left brain as the receiver for Binah (cognitive understanding). So what receives Da'at, the deepest form of eureka-instantaneous-knowing? Remember the eye we imagined at the back of our heads during rooting? Imagine that this spiritual third eye is connected to a third non-physical *triasphere*. It's where we perceive and grasp higher knowledge instantaneously. Perhaps it's in that triasphere that we experience the peek/peak experience.

Finding Meaning

Because the prefix hemi (as in hemisphere) literally means half, I've coined the word **triasphere** to describe the third receiving part of the energy mind. Don't run to Google it; you won't find it.

I believe that when we achieve ocular divergence, and the two hemispheres go to time-out, we can utilize the third triasphere. We can hear the still, small voice that's usually drowned out by all the noise of the other two hemispheres in our minds. Then we can access the wisdom contained higher up within our energy matrix, and from the WEB itself.

Exercises for Ocular Divergence

Now that we understand what ocular divergence is, let's discuss how to do it. The basic skills are simple to learn but take some practice to master.

Start by holding your hands together at arm's length in front of you, with the index fingers touching.

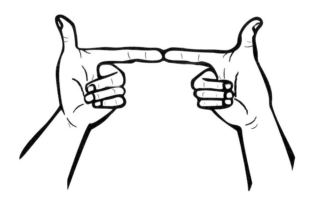

Ocular Divergence: Two fingers touching.

Make sure there's nothing distracting in the background. A clear wall will do nicely. Focus your attention on the point where the fingers meet.

Now very slowly draw your hands closer to you until they're about 6 inches from your eyes. Don't make any effort to keep them in focus. Rather, look through them or past them to see the wall or floor beyond. When your hands are close to your eyes, you'll notice an interesting optical illusion: the appearance of a little "hot dog" floating between your fingers. If you were to separate your fingers a quarter of an inch, this little hot dog would actually float between your fingers.

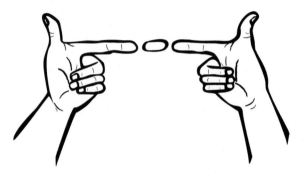

Ocular Divergence: Two fingers separate; floating hot dog.

Once you can see this illusion, you can play with it to improve your skill. First, angle the fingers so they're at a 90-degree angle from each other. The shape of the superbly suspended sausage has now changed to a small heart.

With a little practice, you'll be able to do this quickly and easily. Don't stare; it's all right to blink, though. Relax and daydream at the fingers, remembering to breathe evenly at a 4:4 rate.

You can even see this effect with one finger. Hold up your index finger 6–12 inches from your face. If you look directly at your finger, you'll see just the one finger, but if you look past it at a distant wall or object, you'll see two, floating there like goalposts. What you're actually seeing, as you look past the finger, is what each eye sees independently, one to the left, one to the right.

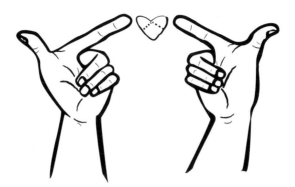

Ocular Divergence: Angled fingers; floating heart.

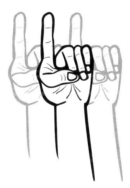

Ocular Divergence: hold up one finger and see two.

Practice shifting back and forth between these two perspectives; from looking *at* the finger to looking *past* the finger, from seeing one finger to seeing two. In this manner, you can teach yourself to achieve ocular divergence.

Reading Between the Lines for Exams

MISC.

If you use this exercise while you study or take an exam, you can relax your mind enough to have better recall of the material. How can you see the material with your finger in the way? Simple: read between the lines. That is, in ocular divergence you can read a book *between* the goalposts of your two fingers.

The last exercise we'll learn can be done with any of the examples already mentioned, but we'll use the last one—one finger, looking like two fingers—as an example.

Hold up your index finger and view it divergently (that is, so you can see both fingers). Once you have the two fingers in your sight, practice closing your eyes for a few seconds and then opening them immediately afterward. See if you can hold the ocular divergence with your eyes closed.

This is very useful for any kind of closed-eyed meditative technique because it enhances your control over the left-right hemispheres uncoupling. If you sense a gentle humming of vibration behind your closed eyes when practicing these exercises, don't worry. It's probably one of your body's natural 8 hz metronomes, helping you to lock into and stay in an alpha state.

I said earlier that you'd been practicing these exercises all your life and I meant it. When you stare out the window at a distant scene, you naturally fall into a daydream state. That's why daydreaming is so relaxing. You've slowed your brain waves down to an alpha state or light trance. The wider the horizon at which you gaze, the easier it is to go into trance.

Have you ever been driving for a long time on a relatively empty road and begun to zone out, then snapped out of it just seconds before you missed your exit? The reason is simple: your eyes locked onto the two painted lines on the road, one eye to each line. Because you weren't looking at either line but rather gazing far down the road in front of you, you naturally fell into ocular divergence. The hemispheres were on time-out, but they were still working. They saw your exit coming—I'm guessing it was the logical, rational brain that did the job—and snapped you back into a conscious beta reality (15–30 hz waking-state brain wave).

stay Grounded   Going into ocular divergence while driving isn't a good idea. Keep your eyes converged when driving and save your trance states for when you aren't moving at 65 mph!

Once you've become fairly competent at achieving ocular divergence, use it as you prepare to practice rooting. As you begin your 4:4 breathing, before the rooting, go into ocular divergence. Then hold on to the divergence as you allow your eyes to close. You'll find it easier to relax.

Ancient and Modern Practices for Ocular Divergence

Meditative and religious systems have made use of this principle for millennia. Here are some examples from the three systems we learned about: yoga, t'ai chi, and Kabbalah.

Yoga

There are two very well-known examples of ocular divergence in yoga. The first is sitting in a meditative posture. Even though you're resting your hands on your knees with your fingers in a specific position known as a *mudra,* you've been told to gaze either at the tip of your nose or upward between your eyebrows. Either way, your eyes are aware of your hands on your knees because they can see your hands peripherally. Presto—you're in divergence.

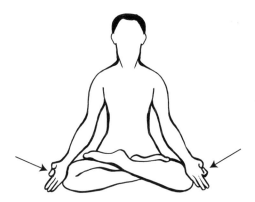

Sitting Posture: Hands cause ocular divergence.

A second example is viewing a *yantra,* a geometrical design that has a deeper symbolic meaning. Because there are no single points to gaze at within the repetitive patterns, your eyes will gaze at the entire yantra, seeing the whole design. You could also gaze at the whole star of David or the cross and have their eyes drawn out to peripheral points. Once again, you're in ocular divergence.

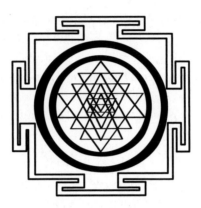

An example of a yantra.

Finding
Meaning

A **mudra** is a physical gesture, done mostly with the hands but can also be a whole body posture. The mudra has spiritual or energy significance in yoga, Hinduism, or Buddhism. When you close your fingers during rooting, it is a mudra.

A **yantra** is a visual focal point for the meditator, just as a mantra is an auditory focal point. Each encourages the meditator to focus on the vibrations of that particular "device." Viewing a yantra meditatively invariably guides you into ocular divergence.

T'ai Chi

The opening move of most styles of t'ai chi is a bowing in by the practitioner, with the body in a very relaxed state. As the body sinks, the hands begin to draw upward to the shoulders and then float back and down, just as you practiced in the Qi Gung rooting exercises in Chapter 14. You don't watch each of the hands going up and down, you view them both peripherally. The wider your peripheral field of vision, the quicker and deeper you go into the ocular divergence zone conducive to the practice of t'ai chi … and energy healing.

Every martial arts class that deals with the subject of street defense will, to some extent, teach you about peripheral vision. You want to use your warrior's radar to sense danger before you become its victim.

In the classic film *The Seven Samurai*, there's a wonderful scene where an endangered town is auditioning samurais—great warriors who live according to bushido, the highly ethical way of the warrior—to defend it from invading gangs. They ask each samurai to go into a building, where a villager is hiding inside the door, waiting to attack him. If the samurai doesn't sense the danger before he's hit, he's immediately disqualified. They all definitely need ocular divergence to succeed. (I won't spoil one of the very funny moments in that scene; rent the DVD and watch it; it's a classic!)

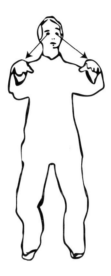

Standing T'ai Chi posture.

Kabbalah

There are many examples of focal points for ocular divergence in Kabbalah, the most famous popularized by Steven Spielberg in *Raiders of the Lost Ark*.

The ark of the covenant was the golden box that held the actual stone tablets on which Moses carved the Ten Commandments. At the top of the ark were two golden cherubs, facing away from each other. The High Priest was the only person allowed into the holy of holies to stand before the ark. Tradition tells us that the High Priest heard the still, small voice of God from between the outstretched wings; not the wings themselves, but from the empty space between them. Jewish tradition also teaches that the High Priest went through a series of intense preparations before entering the holy of holies. You can be certain that his two hemispheres were as diverged as they could get! That helped open what I've called his third triasphere, preparing him to receive the prophecy from as high up on the ladder as he could climb. The sound from the space between the wings of the cherubs was heard in the triasphere between the two hemispheres of his brain.

A 3-D Viewing Exercise

One of the wonders of computer technology is called a stereogram. When I first started using these elegant tools to teach ocular divergence, they weren't well known. Now, everywhere I turn I see Magic Eye books, by far the most advanced of these images anywhere. Once you learn to perform ocular divergence, you'll have no trouble seeing and enjoying these 3-D images. But don't forget why we're learning to do this: when you're in ocular divergence, the brain wave slows down, moving to the 8 hz frequency that allows you to access your energy matrix more easily, log on to the earth and WEB, and then phase-lock with the patient. The 3-D images just make learning it a little more fun!

Look at the illustration. What do you see? Just a random design? Try looking at it another way … literally. All you have to do is go into ocular divergence and you'll be able to see the hidden 3-D image. Here's how. Hold up the picture in front of you, just as you did earlier to see the phenomenal flying franks. Make sure you rotate the book so the two square dots are on the top.

Hold the center of the image right up to your nose. It should be blurry. Focus as though you're looking past the image into the distance. Very slowly move the image away from your face until the two squares above the image turn into three squares. If you see four squares, you may have gone too far or not far enough. Just keep playing until you see three squares, the middle one being the darkest of the three. Now, holding the page still, gaze divergently at the whole page at once. The hidden image will magically appear. It will develop before your eyes like a photograph in a developing tray. The longer you look, the clearer the illusion becomes.

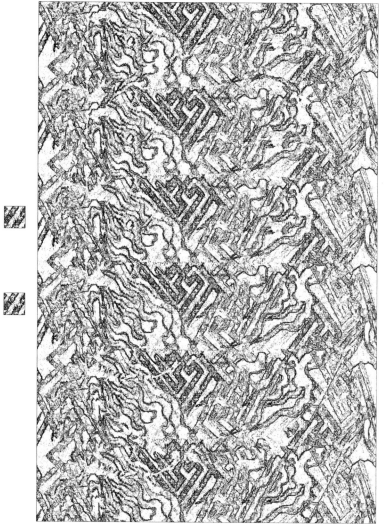

Magic Eye Stereogram exercise.

(Image © 2011 Magic Eye Inc., used with permission.)

If that doesn't work easily, try this second method. Hold the image very close to your nose, so that the whole page is blurred. Forget the dots on top and gaze at the whole page, with your nose aimed at the center of the image. Slowly, keeping the page as steady as possible, draw the picture back away from you. Move very slowly, no more than an inch a second. When they get it somewhere between 6 and 12 away, most people will begin to see the page appear to vibrate or move. Go about an inch more and stop. Continue to gaze at the whole page until the picture begins to surface. Be patient; it takes a few minutes for some people, but once you get it, you'll have no trouble the next time.

This simple piece of art can be used for your daily day-gazing practice instead of using your fingers.

Viewing an Aura

Now that you've read about rooting and ocular divergence, you may want to try seeing an aura. Try having someone sit opposite you, quietly, in front of a clear wall. Go into ocular divergence, directing your gaze both to the left and right sides of his head simultaneously, left eye to the left side, right eye to the right. Keep your gaze steady; don't look back and forth. You may discover that you can see the first level of the aura.

Auditory and Olfactory Divergence

Ocular divergence is the simplest, most common induction into an 8 hz state. However, sight isn't the only sense you can use to induce a light trance. You can also do it through your senses of smell and hearing. The right and left ears are also connected to the two hemispheres, as are the two nostrils. In yoga breathing, you may have encountered the phenomenon that there is usually one nostril that's clearer than the other. This tends to indicate hemisphere dominance as well. For example, if the left nostril is clear, the right hemisphere will be more active, and vice versa. A whole system of yoga, swara yoga, developed to make use of that fact. If a student is taking a math test and needs strong analytic thinking, she's advised to do certain breathing exercises to activate left-brain dominance. Amazingly, lying down on your left side will clear your right nostril, which will send energy to the left brain, improving analytic performance.

The equivalence of divergence through the nose, which we might call olfactory divergence, is what is known as the ujjayi breath in hatha yoga. The word itself means ocean and got its name because of the rushing sound you hear inside your head as you breathe, which comes from the position of the glottis. When you're performing the even breath you learned in Chapter 13, you should be breathing through both nostrils, equally and simultaneously, which is the basic ujjayi breath.

If you'd like to get a clear sense of that ocean sound, perform an even breath while covering your ears. If you're controlling the breath from the diaphragm and flaring the nostrils as you inhale back and down into the throat, you'll hear the same rushing sound you do when you listen to a seashell.

You can modify the even breath by exhaling through the nose, instead of using the "hah" whisper exhalation through the mouth. Try to keep that ocean sound as steady as you can. You'll hear the ocean sound inside your head at the upper center.

As for the ears, what I'd call auditory divergence, is an exercise in focused listening. With a little practice, you can learn to focus your hearing. The next time you listen to an orchestra or choir, try focusing your attention on one instrumentalist or singer. You'll find you can hear them more loudly or more clearly. The next time you're at a party, see if you can focus on one person across the room and hear her voice more clearly (but no eavesdropping, please!). Parents do this all the time at school performances, when they want to hear their child above all others.

In therapeutic hypnosis, there's a technique that involves two hypno-therapists speaking something completely different into each ear of the client, both at the same time. It's called a double induction. Once the therapists determine whether the client's model is more visual, auditory, or kinesthetic, each one tailors his words with images that are appropriate for the hemisphere of the brain he's addressing: speaking through one ear to the cognitive and analytic left brain and speaking through the other ear to the creative, intuitive right brain. It's a very powerful method of inducing a trance state and can even be done with specially designed stereo hypnosis recordings.

misc.

Try Them All at Once

Try doing all three types of divergence at the same time. Begin to breathe a 4:4 breath in ocular divergence. Focus on breathing through both nostrils. Imagine extending your hearing outwardly with each ear like radar, as if searching for sounds on either side of the room. Simultaneously, feel the breath inside your head and listen inwardly with your third ear to the ocean rush sound of the breath. The effect of this exercise is quite powerful.

Essential Takeaways

- Ocular divergence is found in most ancient systems of meditation to help induce a light trance state, utilizing different visual focal points depending on the culture.

- By practicing the simple exercises in this chapter, you can train the brain to enter an uncoupled–hemisphere state easily and quickly.

- Practice these exercises often; they can be very effective in developing your skills of energy healing.

- The same principles can be applied for auditory and olfactory divergence, which will similarly bring one to an 8 hz state more easily, conducive for energy healing.

chapter 16

Cleansing the Energy Matrix Through Self-Massage

Using the Reflex Balance (RB) technique

Thumb tips and tricks for self-massage

The RB everyday areas

Self-massage is a time-tested method for cleansing and balancing the energy matrix. Its purpose is to help the body's own self-healing systems function at peak efficiency. There are many techniques and systems available to accomplish this. I've chosen RB or Reflex Balance; it is a system that I began to research and develop almost 40 years ago and I have found it to be a simple, efficient way to cleanse the energy matrix.

Reflex Balance

Reflex Balance (RB) is based on the centuries-old technique of massaging the hands and feet for general therapeutic purposes. If we consider the human body and energy matrix to be a hologram—an integrally related functioning whole in which every part is totally connected to every other part—then theoretically any one part of the system can download or receive information from the whole energy matrix and upload information back to it. In RB you use the feet and hands as holographic access systems to balance the entire energy matrix.

Starting from Scratch

MISC.

After years of collecting and analyzing every zone therapy and reflexology chart I could find, amassing quite a library in the process, I discovered inconsistencies, omissions, and even the occasional absurdity. Certain errors in logic were passed down from one incarnation of reflexology chart to the next, apparently without anyone catching the problems. My approach was to gut the whole thing and start over from the beginning. The result was RB.

I've always felt that if we had the right techniques to practice, and the right attitude, we could enhance our well-being immeasurably. The reason most of us don't feel 100 percent all the time is that we neither choose, nor use, the techniques.

Since the 1970s I've researched and tested the premise of the holographic access system as I developed RB and refined it further and further. I wanted to develop the best possible system of palpation of the feet and hands, one that would meet the high standards I'd been looking for in other systems. My goal was to do the following:

- Create maps of the organs, systems, and structures of the body to be charted with anatomical accuracy.

- Incorporate both the meridians of t'ai chi healing and the chakras of yoga to those maps.

- Incorporate some of the additional complex energy inter-connections from those two systems, including the five-element theory of t'ai chi healing and Puharich's 30-year study on the physics of the chakras.

- Incorporate psycho-emotional and psycho-spiritual imbalances into the arena of what RB could deal with.

- Simplify everything, so patients could learn how to do it for themselves, by incorporating breathing, rooting, and ocular divergence into the self-massage protocol.

- Find an objective way of measuring changes in the body or energy matrix, beyond what a patient might tell me subjectively.

- Develop a detailed diagnostic protocol that incorporated multi-level scanning (see Chapter 17), pulses, and palpation. All three together would enable more precise isolation of the cause of the problem on the proper frequency within the energy matrix.

I began with some basics. To test the hypothesis that the feet or hands are a holographic access system to the energy matrix, I started with a simple cause-and-effect approach. I wanted to be able to press a point on the feet or hands that's related to a particular organ—the stomach, let's say—to see if it could tell me something about a stomachache the patient was experiencing. I used the universally accepted principle in energy healing that if a point is tender, it's the body telling me that something is wrong or out of balance in the energy matrix related to that point.

I would then palpate that point more fully, sending a message back to the stomach to relax. If the stomachache disappeared, that was good—but obviously subjective. If the healing time was faster than expected, that was also a good sign. It would help confirm the premise that we have established a two-way communication with the energy matrix through the holographic access systems of the feet or hands.

Although many other parts of the body can be used in this manner, the hands and feet are ideal. Their surfaces are large enough to work on with ease and precision, yet they are easily accessible and small enough for each person to work on himself.

Palpating Soft Tissue

MISC.

Not every palpation point that's tender is indicative of an energy imbalance. Sometimes there's a physical bruise in an area, or arthritic tenderness causing the discomfort. Also, putting pressure on a bone that's close to the skin will get a painful response from the nearby nerves. With experience, you can learn to palpate soft tissue with moderate pressure and detect energy imbalances.

The years of testing paid off: RB developed to meet my initial goals and even exceed some of them. Many of the case-related successes in this book were accomplished through the use of RB. Yet with all the complex material synthesized into the system, I consider the most important accomplishment the development of the everyday areas, a simple and basic massage protocol that each person can do on her own hands and feet. In 5 to 10 minutes daily, you can balance your energy matrix and help promote self-healing.

While there's a professional level of RB for training practitioners, my focus in this chapter is to teach you the everyday areas for general balancing of your energy matrix. These are things you can do for yourself. If you're already a trained healer, your balanced energy matrix makes you a better channel for the energy that flows through you to your patient.

stay Grounded

There's a natural temptation to discount anything that seems too simple. If I taught you all kinds of complex reflex points related to RB meridians and chakras, you might be more inclined to work on those than on the simple shaded areas on the everyday areas chart. Don't be fooled! Simple is not simplistic. These everyday areas are simple to do, but their results can be profound. Keep it simple!

Your job will be to palpate, or massage, in a press-and-roll drilling motion, all the shaded or darkened areas on the following charts. It will only take a few minutes each day. Think of it in the same way you think of brushing your teeth. If you brush and floss every day, you'll generally avoid a lot of serious dental problems. If something more serious comes up, then you can go to the dentist (or the energy healer, in this analogy) to deal with it.

RB Everyday Self-Massage

Let's start with the everyday areas of RB. These are the points that stimulate the body's own control systems and help you stay well. Once you've learned the technique, these are the areas you'll want to work every day.

For those who are curious about which areas within the body's energy matrix you're balancing through the RB-holographic access system, I've included a list of the corresponding organs, glands, muscles, etc., to each shaded area.

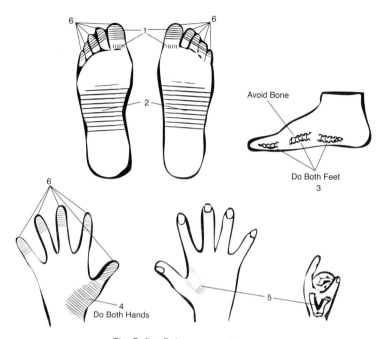

The Reflex Balance everyday areas.

These simple shaded diagrams include RB points for the following organs and systems:

1. The big toe: pituitary, pineal, hypothalamus, thalamus, basal nuclei, medulla and cerebellum, assorted meridians, and the fifth, sixth, and seventh chakras. Also, palpate the shaded area at the base of the big toe (on the top of the ball of the foot) for the thyroid and parathyroid glands.

2. Arch of foot: gastrointestinal and genitourinary tract, adrenals, ovaries/testes, rectum, uterus/prostate, assorted meridians, and the first, second, and third chakras.

3. Inside edge of foot: spinal column, the nervous system, and assorted meridians.

4. Thumb base (also called the thenar eminence): lungs, thymus, thyroid, parathyroid, heart and pericardium, assorted meridians, and the fourth and fifth chakras.

5. The *hoku* area (the rim of the web on the back of your hands): thalamus, hypothalamus, basal nuclei, medulla oblongata, and the pituitary and pineal glands, and the fifth, sixth, and seventh chakras.

Finding Meaning

The **hoku** point (also pronounced hegu) is a powerful acupuncture point that lies along the large intestine meridian. It's best known as a headache point. The hoku is called tiger jaw because of the position of the metacarpals, or bones, that frame it. In RB, when I refer to the hoku area, I'm talking about the entire area along both bone ridges as shown in the diagram.

6. Padded tips of fingers and toes: brain, midbrain, cranial nerves, sensory organs, sinuses, and assorted meridians.

Before you go running off to massage these areas, read through the technique section. That way you'll get the most out of it.

The Technique of Palpation-Massage

The following "rules of thumb" should give you a crash course in how to practice RB on yourself.

As you prepare to do the RB everyday areas on yourself, try to practice some of the breathing, rooting, or ocular divergence skills you've learned, just to get into a "healing" frame of mind. If you practice other forms of grounding or breathing techniques, use the system you're comfortable with.

1. Always begin by washing your hands. This isn't just for sanitary purposes but also to cleanse your hands for energy healing.

2. Place the tip of your thumb (not the flat pad or fingerprint of the thumb) on the RB point you wish to palpate. You want to cover the entire surface of any shaded area in the illustration.

3. Begin by inhaling for two counts. As you drill into the point in a circular fashion, exhale for four counts. If the RB point is tender, repeat the palpation with a 2:4 breath (inhale 2: exhale 4) to the

same point a second time. If the RB point isn't tender or painful, move on to the next point until you've completed palpating all of the shaded or darkened areas on the chart.

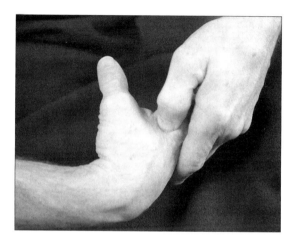

Thumb position in palpation.

4. Be sure to do these same points every day until the tenderness goes away. This may take days, weeks, even months. The body heals in its own time. Once these points are balanced, check them regularly for disease prevention. The check only takes a few seconds per reflex each day. If the point starts to become tender again, increase the length of time you apply pressure.

5. The 2:4 breath is a composite of two breaths. Inhale briskly as in a 2:2 pacing breath, and exhale more slowly, as in a 4:4 even breath.

6. Don't overdo. Two 2:4 breaths are sufficient for any tender point. Remember that 5 to 10 a day is better than once a week for an hour. Be gentle with yourself at first. Tomorrow's always another day.

7. Always maintain an even breathing pattern as you work the reflexes. Correct breathing will help you handle the tenderness you may feel at certain reflexes.

Both breathing and rooting help to release the toxic energy released by massage. We don't want to free up energy plaque and then re-circulate it into the system. Breathe and root it away.

8. Keep your eyes open. Even if you've learned about deep breathing with eyes closed, keeping your eyes open during an RB session will prevent hyperventilation and help you concentrate your attention on the balancing-healing process. Because you live with your eyes open, take responsibility for your health the same way: with your eyes open.

9. If your thumb doesn't have sufficient strength for palpation, you can augment it with the other thumb, as in the photographs.

10. You'll have to cut long fingernails, at least on your thumbs. If you aren't willing to do that at first, use the rubber eraser at the tip of a pencil, though your personal energy will be much better.

11. Don't practice RB immediately before or after a big meal or heavy exercise. Don't practice RB under the immediate influence of medications or alcohol. Be especially gentle if you suffer from diabetes, heart disease, blood pressure disorders, or any problem that requires medical monitoring. Also be especially gentle when working on the hands or feet during pregnancy or if you're trying to become pregnant.

12. Remember that chronic problems take longer to balance than acute problems. Be patient and persevere when practicing RB.

13. In working on muscular or joint pain, be prepared for an occasional intensification of the pain before it improves, usually in the first 24 to 48 hours after the session. This is caused by the body's acceleration of the healing process. The pain will soon pass and you'll feel better than before. RB won't make any pain permanently worse.

14. Remember that you aren't treating anything; you're balancing the energy field of the body, thereby helping it heal itself. Approach this balancing process with care and gentleness. Try to practice RB in a quiet, well-ventilated place at the same time every day. Relax yourself with breathing techniques and rooting before you start. Concentrate on what you're doing. Wash your hands before and after each session.

Sitting in the right position to massage your own feet can be challenging. The basic sitting positions are either on the floor or on the edge of a bed or chair. Choose the one most comfortable for you. A good time to work on your feet is in the morning before you get out of bed.

I can't emphasize enough how important it is to palpate these areas every day. The results will be best with a long-term approach. Don't just massage a point to get rid of a symptom. Do all the areas every day to keep the energy matrix as balanced as possible.

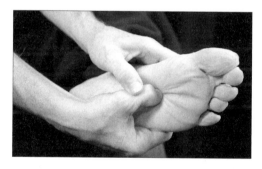

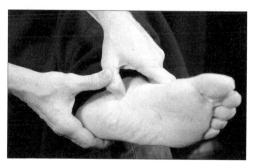

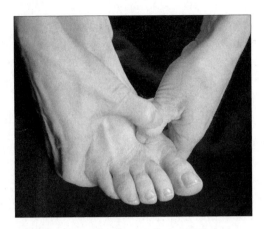

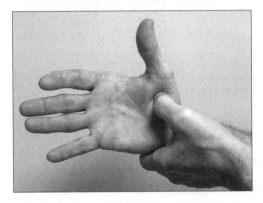

Examples of how to do the everyday areas.

Essential Takeaways

- RB is a modern system developed by the author to cleanse the energy matrix by using palpation of the feet and hands.
- While the system is fairly complex, the everyday areas are simple enough for you to apply for yourself with great benefit.
- Use your breathing to deal with any initial discomfort caused by the RB, and to cleanse the body of any energy plaque that's released during the massage.
- Pay attention to the rules of thumb to get the most out of the palpation, and to make sure you're doing it safely.

chapter 17

Scanning the Energy Matrix

One of the most direct ways of detecting and gathering information from the energy matrix concerning health or imbalances within the body is the ability to scan it with your hands. This is a trainable technique, but it generally takes time, practice, and a teacher's guidance to master.

Diagnosing and Treating the Energy Matrix

Once a healer's energy matrix is properly grounded with the rooting process or an equivalent, she'll be able to safely sense the patient's energy field with relative ease. But the fact that a healer can feel energy in her hands doesn't mean she can understand or interpret what she feels. Just because I can see the squiggles on an EEG doesn't mean I understand what they mean.

I once met a young man who had been deaf from birth and had just gotten a cochlear implant that enabled him to hear sounds for the first time. He could finally hear, but he couldn't yet understand the random sounds he heard. He said it would take months to train his brain to process language well enough to carry on basic communication. In the same way, once a healer learns to sense energy fields, patience and training are then required to learn how to process the new information.

Learning Patience

When I first learned to feel energy with my teacher, I was in a hurry to do something with it. I was told to be patient. I was taught that it was important to get to the point where what I felt was actually there, and not something I was just guessing at. My teacher would place an object before me and ask me to describe the energy I felt coming from it. Then she would tell me what she felt. It took a while before I felt the same thing she did, but it did happen eventually.

The challenge in scanning is to ask a question and then silence the mind as completely as possible to await an answer. That may sound simple, but it isn't. We all have a knowledge base within us that anticipates an answer before it comes. Ironically, the more experienced the healer, the greater the database of information she has, and therefore the less likely it is that she'll be able to quiet her mind and listen for what the patient's energy matrix has to say.

Many systems use different methods of scanning to read the energy matrix. For those of you who are new to energy healing, I'll describe what happens in a basic session with a patient. Please note that this is presented as one person's example of energy matrix scanning. It isn't offered as the definitive way that this is done in every system, nor is it a lesson for you to try on someone else. Be patient, follow along, and take in the basic lessons that follow.

The Scanning Process

I always wash my hands to disperse any vibrations from other people or objects I might have touched and then root (or ground myself) at the deepest possible level I can. Once the patient is lying comfortably and quietly on the table, I help him initiate a 4:4 breathing rhythm. As I guide him into this relaxed state, I place my hand above his head with the intention to entrain or phase-lock with his energy matrix.

I float my other hand slowly over his body in a descending path over his chakras. I empty my mind and try to listen-feel the energy; listening is a passive process, while feeling is an active one. When scanning, we have to do both. Quiet the mind and be passive, but don't just sit there and wait for the energy to come to you. Seek it out. If I were drawing what I feel, it would be a kind of wavy line, like a sound wave, or a sine curve in algebra. There will be ups and downs as I pass directly over the chakras and the spaces between. I do this several times until I feel completely in tune with the patient's energy matrix.

The Chakra Locations

The location of each of the chakras is very close to a specific endocrine gland and neurological plexus, as indicated in the table in Chapter 2. Once you're familiar with the chakras, you don't really think about those positions during the scan, only the feel of each one.

By the fourth pass, I'm usually ready to pay attention to the pattern of his unique energy matrix. Having done this so many times, I know what a generally healthy wave should feel like, so I immediately recognize anything that might depart from that pattern. The most obvious things I look for are the energy highs and lows—places where I feel a surge or deficiency of energy. Then I look for subtler distinctions. The language used to describe what I feel sounds a bit outlandish, but it's similar to the distinctions that t'ai chi healers and doctors use when they utilize the Chinese pulse system for diagnosis: cold/hot, smooth/prickly, moist/dry, hard/soft and puffy, full/empty, floating/sunken, etc.

As mentioned earlier, traditional texts in acupuncture list 28 of the most common qualities of pulses, but clearly there are many more. To the beginner, these can sound very subjective, but in time, a well-trained healer can derive a remarkable amount of information from this apparently simple process of scanning.

Don't worry if this sounds a bit esoteric. To understand this clearly, you really have to experience it. In addition, different healers may experience different sensations. With training, they can learn to interpret what they feel.

Once I've targeted the areas I feel are out of balance through the scanning, I proceed to work on them with focused energy, massage, breath, and, of course, intent.

Intention: The Art of Aiming the Mind

Intention is an essential and fundamental tool for the energy healer. Just as it requires intent to lift your arm by activating neurons and muscles, so the movement of energy in healing requires intent. Energy healing doesn't happen without the expressed intention of the healer, first to attune to their own energy matrix, then to attune to the WEB, and finally to phase-lock with the energy matrix of the patient to facilitate the flow of healing energy.

As I mentioned in Chapter 7, there is a Hebrew word for intention: kavana. It comes from the Hebrew root "kĕʾvūn" which means aim or direction. It is considered indispensible to prayer and meditation. The renowned mystic master, Rabbi Abraham Isaac Kook, states: "Kavana is everything. The revival of kavana is the revival of the world … every act that perfects the world is embraced in it."

Every system of energy healing has its own methodology for training intention. It can begin with something as simple as counting the duration of each inhalation and exhalation. Or it could involve training in ocular divergence, reciting a mantra, gazing at a yantra, doing mindfulness meditation, playing an instrument, or doing a T'ai Chi form. Any and all of these are valid. Intent is the least tangible and perhaps the most essential tool for energy healing.

Regardless of how you train for it, I believe that proper intent requires three basic qualities: disciplined spiritual imagination.

- Intent requires that the mind is disciplined enough to be silent when you need it to be, allowing you to hear that still, small voice within.

- Intent must be spiritually directed for its use in energy healing, though it will also impact many other endeavors including playing an instrument, engaging in a sport, designing a new app, or presenting a case before a jury.

- With regard to intent and energy healing, imagination doesn't refer to making something up, but rather the ability to hold an image still and focused in the mind, without expectation or agenda.

It is fair to say that any system of energy healing that does not include the subject of intent in the training protocol will be the poorer for it.

Basic Training in Energy Scanning

A complete method of scanning is quite intricate and beyond the scope of this book, but here are some basic exercises that will give you a sense of how it works and feels.

Let's start with an inanimate object rather than a person. Every object has a vibratory signature, and we've already learned that water, crystals, and other objects have a memory, so let's try to scan some of them and see if we can access some feeling or information. Remember, you have to crawl before you walk and walk before you run. When I first began my studies in acupuncture, we learned how to insert needles into oranges and bananas. That was fine, until I found out that the first person I had to needle was myself!

A good object to start with is a simple quartz crystal. If you don't have one handy, you can use a precious or semi-precious jewel (diamond, emerald, sapphire, opal, amethyst, jade, etc.).

1. Wash your hands. This is both a physical washing and a ritual energy cleansing. Obviously, if your hands are dirty, you should wash them thoroughly first; then take a moment to imagine dispersing any toxic energy you may have been in contact with.

2. Breathe for a few minutes; use the fast/slow breathing set you learned in Chapter 13. That will pump up your energy in the first half and quiet you down in the second, slower half. It establishes a calm state of energy equilibrium conducive to scanning.

3. Now take a few minutes to root. Follow that with the energy biofeedback Qi Gung technique outlined in Chapter 14, so you have a tingling sensation in your hands (hot or cold or magnetic push-or-pull).

4. Hold the crystal or whatever object you're using in your right hand, pointing upward.

5. With your left hand, begin to pass over the stone very slowly from right to left. When you've gone beyond the crystal by 4 to 6 inches, circle back toward yourself (counterclockwise) and begin again. Don't go back over the stone in the opposite direction.

6. After three or four passes be attentive to what you feel as you're directly over the stone.

7. Finally, hold your hand over the stone without moving and find the hot spot, the position where whatever you feel is strongest. It could be pushing upward or pulling downward. Don't try to outguess what you think the sensation should be. Keep your mind as empty as possible, as if you've asked a question and are awaiting an answer. See what you get.

8. Wash your hands.

If you're having trouble visualizing this process, turn to the Resources appendix for information on helpful videos.

If you're working with a partner, the two of you can test your diagnostic accuracy. Using the principle of Dr. Emoto's water crystals, take two small bottles of distilled water and label them A and B. Write a positive phrase on one piece of paper and a negative phrase on the other. Have your partner place a bottle on top of each message, and then leave them for 24 hours. Don't peek! Only your partner will know which bottle was absorbing the energy of which message. The next day, with the paper removed, repeat the scanning steps listed above. See if you can feel which is which. It's sort of the energy counterpart of the famous Coke/Pepsi Challenge.

Try Not to Influence Each Other

If you're practicing scanning objects with a friend, don't tell him what you felt until he's tried it, too. Then compare what you each got to see if they're similar. Try using several types of stones to see if you can sense a difference.

You don't want to go too far without a teacher, but now you can try a simple version of scanning a person. When someone has an ache or pain and she asks you for help, go through the eight basic training steps. When you reach the seventh step, hold your hand over the most intense spot, which may or may not be exactly where she feels the pain. Send a positive healing thought to that hot spot with the intention to balance her energy to help the energy matrix heal itself. Because you're rooted, imagine the earth's energy flowing through you to the patient's energy matrix. You're simply a channel and aren't using your own energy, just providing the right intention.

Keep your mind clear, allowing the energy to flow through you. You may or may not feel some sensation. After a moment or two, re-scan. If it feels better to you, thank the patient for allowing you to be of help. If you sense a little more energy is needed, repeat the scanning technique, find the hot spot, which may not be in exactly the same place as before, and project your healing intention again. Then wash your hands. You're done for now.

Scanning can be done in many ways. A friend of mine, Dr. John Shisler, chose to become a full-time dowser later in life. He taught many methods, using dowsing rods, pendulums, and other devices. The device itself isn't important; it's the state of mind the dowser is in as he asks the question and waits for the yes/no answer that matters. If the mind isn't clear, the device won't do anything.

First the dowser or scanner programs the device to respond to a question with a specific action that can be clearly identified as a yes or a no. For example, a yes answer might make the free-hanging pendulum spin clockwise; a negative response would make it spin counter-clockwise. Once that's established, she uses the pendulum as a focal point when asking a question, for example, "Is there a deep water well here?" The answer to the yes/no question is based on which way the pendulum spins.

Deeper connections

My mother-in-law once told me that when she was a child in Romania, it was common to see farmers dowse eggs to see which ones had been fertilized and were going to become chickens. I've also seen energy healers dowse expectant mothers for the gender of their fetus. In all cases, it's not the pendulum or the dowsing rods that matter; it's the state of mind of the dowser.

I watched Dr. Shisler as he dowsed for water pipes and wells. He claimed his success rate was over 90 percent. He also searched for what he called geopathic zones, which were places on the planet that seemed to have a negative energy around them. People who lived over these underground zones—blockages in the earth's energy matrix—had become ill with similar diseases, often years apart. He tried to re-route the zones with giant stakes he put into the earth at different locations. It seemed to me like doing acupuncture to the planet, just as he might have placed needles balancing excess or deficient energy in the meridians.

I recall one strange case of this kind of locational, rather than human, scanning. A woman called me and said she'd bought a condo in Miami. She was having it renovated, and everything that could go wrong was going wrong. Glass was breaking, tiles were cracking, paint was chipping away instead of holding to the walls, and workers were suffering all sorts of accidental injuries. There also seemed to be problems with the appliances that were being delivered. She wanted to know if I could do something to "heal" her apartment. It was way out of my skill-set. It sounded more like a case for the Ghostbusters! I really had no idea what to do, but I said I'd give it a try. I entered the condo alone and walked around a bit, feeling a little out of my element. As I emptied my mind and rooted, it occurred to me to scan each room to see if I felt anything. Everything was pretty normal until I got to one particular room. The energy there was intense, out of balance, and almost painful in my scanning hand. I intensified my breathing and directed my intentions to break up the negative energy and balance, whatever it was.

Three days later, the woman called to tell me that everything seemed to be better. Nothing had gone wrong since I'd been there. Then she said she'd checked with the building manager and found out that the elderly woman who'd previously owned the condo had died in the room in which I'd felt the strange energy. Because she lived alone, her body hadn't been found for several days. Who knows whether her final suffering might not have left an energy imprint on the room? I admit, it sounds like something out of the *Twilight Zone*; I think I can even hear some of you humming the theme song!

Blind Diagnosis at the Medical School

From 1982 to 1984, I conducted a periodic seminar called Alternative Modalities in Family Care Practice at the Bowman Gray School of Medicine at Wake Forest University, intended for third-year medical students. It was a unique opportunity for me to introduce acupuncture and acupressure, and how those modalities work with young doctors. At the end of the program the professor in charge wrote to me the following:

> "The students have particularly appreciated demonstrations of the diagnostic and therapeutic potential of these methods. Certainly the most important aspect of your presentation is the challenge to open our minds to some of the capabilities we may possess that are not well explained by our current scientific belief systems. One example has been your 'blind diagnosis' demonstration in which you take the 'Chinese pulses,' palpate a variety of acupuncture points, scan the body with your hand, and then attempt to provide a diagnostic readout of the patient's condition—without benefit of a medical history. The participants have been very impressed with your diagnostic accuracy."

The Deepest Cut of All

Whenever the physical body has surgery, the trauma to the body produces an energy reaction. As the body heals itself from the surgery, the energy matrix should balance and heal, too. Sometimes that "energy scar" remains and causes problems. To prevent such problems, you should routinely balance the energy matrix once the physical body has healed from any surgery.

The blind diagnosis experiment he spoke of began with a challenge from one of the students at the very first class. She said, "If this really works, let's see you diagnose someone, just using your … stuff." The assistant chairman of the department, who was present, volunteered. I took no medical history whatsoever; he simply got on the examination table and lay down.

One has to wonder if any doctor or medical student would ever agree to diagnose a patient without taking a medical history. But, for fun, I accepted the challenge and scanned his body, took his pulses, and palpated a few

RB points. I explained that I wasn't going to label diseases—that was their job—but I would identify where I thought health problems would be found. I went to the chalkboard and wrote down "Sinuses, lower back, duodenum, and groin." When I was done, the man confirmed that he had chronic sinusitis, chronic lower-back problems, a duodenal ulcer, and had undergone a vasectomy six months earlier.

There was quite a buzz in the room. The students decided to promote me from guest lecturer to sorcerer. The following rotation, about six weeks later, the room was crowded with additional professors, including the chairman of the department. Apparently there had been some discussion about how I had "pulled that off."

On my second try, I hit the 100 percent correct mark again and was jokingly promoted from sorcerer to wizard. Each time I held the seminar, the students tried to find people with more and more outlandish problems for me to diagnose. Over a 2-year period and 12 trials, the professor in charge of the program calculated my success rate at 85 percent overall accuracy. It opened some minds and encouraged me to further refine my diagnostic method.

Deeper Connections

In the second case, I wrote "Stomach, right knee, and liver." The doctor did have a stomach ulcer and a right knee scheduled for surgery. I worked on it for about a minute, and the pain seemed to go away. I later learned that the surgery was cancelled. Regarding the liver, he denied any problem. Once he left the room, however, the laughter began; everyone in the room apparently knew he was a drinker. You can't fool all the people (or the energy matrix) all the time.

Two Fascinating Cases

Every person I work with has something to teach. Two cases come to mind as particularly significant in energy scanning, as they pointed me to deeper ideas and discoveries.

The Energy Relationship of Body and Emotions

After years of scanning chakras, I was getting pretty good at discovering physiological disorders. Because each chakra had a glandular and neurological connection, the imbalance on the energy level pointed at a possible problem on the related organic level. If that was so, I reasoned, why not try to map the psycho-emotional relationships that yoga associates with the chakras, to see if they could point to a deeper source or cause of the problem? After much research, I created a tentative map of the psycho-emotional component of the chakras, which served as a doorway, if you will, into the psychological state of the patient. I called the psycho-emotional level "rung 2," with the physiological level called "rung 1."

As always, I asked the patient's permission to entrain his energy matrix for information. I always begin by scanning rung 1, as that's the area I'm more familiar with. Then, as if changing channels on a radio receiver, I ask the energy matrix for information on rung 2. As I scanned, I felt something that seemed subtler but had more or less the same shape. I wasn't immediately overwhelmed by the results, as the patterns seemed so similar.

Then I began to notice something interesting in some of the cases. Every so often, one of the chakras on rung 2 was very different, almost contradictory or opposite, from its counterpart on rung 1. And whenever that happened, it turned out that it was on that chakra's level that the patient's symptoms had occurred.

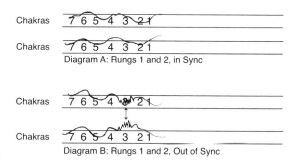

Two examples of Rung 1–2. Scanning: In sync and out of sync.

For example, on the level of the third chakra, when scanning rung 1, I would often find problems related to the digestive or immune systems. On rung 2 of the same chakra, there were issues of the patients being more assertive, or the inability to yield to circumstances in their lives. When the scans of rung 1 and rung 2 were opposite each other at a particular chakra, that would invariably be the level on which the patient was experiencing symptoms and disorders.

Rungs of the energy matrix can directly affect each other. I had a patient who was a bully, always super-asserting himself and never yielding to anyone, even when common sense would suggest he do so. That excess energy on the third chakra on rung 2—the psycho-emotional level— caused a deficiency of energy on the same chakra on rung 1, the physiological level. The result was, he had a very inefficient digestive system that led to chronic constipation and other intestinal problems.

In more conventional terms, it seemed that when the body and emotions were out of sync, the body would manifest symptoms to send a message down the ladder to alert the patient to do something about it. That wasn't surprising in itself. What was amazing to me was that a scan of the energy matrix could yield the information if I asked the right questions. I tried this many times in a blind diagnosis format to be sure I wasn't simply feeling what I expected to feel.

As the years went on, I found that this relationship between the physiological and psycho-emotional provided a wealth of information that enabled me to help patients help themselves, and to achieve a greater success in energy healing. In time, this approach led to a similar development on the psycho-spiritual level (rung 3) and access to a whole new source of causes of energy imbalances and the subsequent potential for deeper energy healing.

On Another Level

Just as the theoretical model for the psycho-emotional level (rung 2) was based on yoga and Chinese sources, the source for the model of the psycho-spiritual (rung 3) level was based on Kabbalistic sources related to the inner-dimensions of the sefirot and the olamot (see Chapter 2).

A Case of Multiple Personalities

One of the most unusual examples of this multi-rung approach to scanning happened a few years later. A psychotherapist I had successfully helped with some simple energy issues of her own asked me if I would see one of her patients concerning stress issues.

The patient seemed a rather friendly, optimistic, sociable young woman with a genial attitude. After we spoke a bit, I put her on the table and scanned her energy matrix. As always, I sketched my findings on a graph designed to record the stronger and weaker chakras.

I scanned the patient and sketched her pattern on the graph. I could see certain erratic highs and lows, as with anyone. I taught her how to do basic breathing and gave her some specific RB points related to what I found, in addition to palpating the everyday areas, and scheduled our next appointment.

When she arrived the following week, she almost seemed to be a different person. She was depressed, tearful, unfriendly, uncooperative, and even unable to make eye contact with me. When I scanned her energy matrix this time, to see if my first balancing and the homework she had done had had any lasting effect, I was floored. There was hardly anything similar to the general pattern I'd seen before. Typically, the overall pattern of the chakras doesn't change much; specific blockages or abnormalities will change, but the energy matrix is like your energy signature, staying fairly consistent throughout your life.

Deeper Connections

The changes and consistencies of the wave form of the chakras are analogous to those of your physical body. From one year to the next, you might change your hair and lose some weight, but even if you look very different, when you run into a friend you haven't seen in a while she'll still know it's you. The chakras are the same way; you can develop or upgrade your chakras, but they still follow the same basic pattern.

Two chakra areas on her new scan, around the mouth and lower abdomen, were off the charts with erratic energy. Those two areas, on the physiological rung 1 level, were also totally out of synch with the psycho-emotional rung 2 pattern. There had been no hint of those imbalances just a week before. I balanced her energy matrix as best I could, gave her some homework exercises, and sent her on her way.

I called her psychotherapist to ask what was going on. I explained that my scan from the second session wasn't recognizable as the same person from the first. The therapist was silent for a moment, and then told me how amazing that was and explained why.

This patient had been diagnosed with dissociative identity disorder, commonly called multiple personality disorder. Each of her different selves seemed to be consciously unaware of the others. When I described her energy pattern at the second session, the therapist said, "Oh, that must have been Eva you were seeing." Apparently Eva was the personality who held memories of sexual abuse (specifically involving the mouth) by a relative, as well as repeated physical abuse to her stomach. Those were the same areas that displayed the greatest energy trauma: the mouth and lower abdomen.

That blew me away. I was aware of the idea of multiple personalities; I'd seen *Sybil* and *The Three Faces of Eve* but assumed that was just exaggerated fiction. It never would have occurred to me that it was real, or that each personality might have a completely different energy profile. I really had seen two different people at the two sessions.

We decided that, with the patient's permission, we'd continue to see whether we could help her. Under hypnosis, the therapist invited the different personalities into the body and I scanned each one to try to balance her. Working with the psychotherapist, we helped her on the path to becoming a more balanced and integrated young woman.

Without question, that was the most startling case of scanning I had ever encountered. It gave me a new perspective and respect for the energy dimensions of our lives. It also reminded me of just how important energy healing can be as a complement to traditional medicine and psychotherapy, and how much more we can accomplish when we work together.

Essential Takeaways

- All things have an energy signature. The key in scanning is tuning in to the right frequency or wavelength.
- In scanning, always prepare yourself, as directed, so you can interact with the energy matrix safely.
- Before you start working on people, first test your accuracy with objects.
- In addition to the physiological, there are psycho-emotional and psycho-spiritual levels within the energy matrix.

Part 4

Lessons from the World of Energy Healing

If you're seeking out an energy healer, how will you determine which modality is right for you? What are the factors that will guide your decision? We'll explore questions that perspective patients can ask to help make informed decisions about energy healing.

We'll also look at some of the things you should know before embarking on the path of becoming an energy healer. As you do your due diligence to select the system that's right for you, we'll arm you with the right questions to give you a solid head start.

It is said that a smart person will learn from his or her own mistakes but a wise person can also learn from someone else's experiences. So we'll conclude our journey in energy healing by looking at some of the lessons learned from a healer's lifetime of work.

Chapter 18

Questions the Energy Healing Patient Should Ask

Doing due diligence in choosing an energy healer

Knowing your responsibilities as a patient

What to expect at an energy healing session

We've talked about the energy healing paradigm, looked at many examples of different systems, and seen a whole array of specific case studies where energy healing was effective. A lot of that was geared toward the aspiring healer, but if you're just looking to become a more educated consumer before visiting an energy healer yourself, here's a guide to help you find the right fit.

Finding the Right Energy Healer

The first decision to make is what type of energy healing is the one for you. As you read through the chapters in Part 2, it's possible you found yourself drawn to one particular system, but if you're still unsure, here are some tools to help you choose.

Is Energy Healing Right for You?

The first thing you'll want to do is assess why you're drawn to energy healing. Let's ask some questions that may focus your intentions.

- Are you afraid of doctors, maybe going all the way back to that first shot during childhood?

- Have you heard horror stories about conventional medicine?

- Have you seen conventional doctors for your problems who've been unable to help you?

- Are you satisfied with what your conventional doctor has been doing but want to complement that treatment with something more holistic?

- Have you gotten a clean bill of health but still feel low on energy, without a full sense of wellness?

- Do you feel your spiritual beliefs are too distant and removed from your day-to-day physical reality?

The answers to all these questions are personal. They reflect your background, history, and paradigm. I want to express one word of caution, though, before you make any drastic choices. If you aren't happy with your doctor, get another one! Don't use energy healing as an either/or alternative to conventional medicine. Both are more effective when they work together. You'd be amazed how many physicians these days are aware of complementary and alternative systems and are, at least in part, sympathetic to some elements of the energy healing world.

Once you've determined why you're looking into energy healing, there are some decisions you'll want to make.

Do you want a gentle laying-on-of-hands healer to help you along? Do you want something a little more physical, involving deep massage, needles, or electro-stimulation? While the idea of being stuck with acupuncture needles may be a bit daunting for some, you'll discover that the needles are pretty benign.

If the healer gives you some homework, how willing are you to follow that advice and undertake a daily regimen to help yourself?

While many healers try to teach their patients skills to help themselves, not every healer is inclined to that approach. Some are more like the energy counterparts of conventional medicine's "treat 'em and street 'em" doctors: you come to see them, they work on you, and you go home.

Are you interested in a short or a long therapy experience? Some people prefer to go to a healer short term, from one to five sessions. If nothing changes in their condition, they move on. At the other extreme, some people are looking for something more long term; one or two times a week for the rest of their lives. In the middle, some systems call for a series of 10 sessions and then another round of 10 if the situation warrants it. That can go on for some time.

I personally prefer about 10 hours total, divided up in 5 to 7 sessions, with a heavy emphasis on what I can teach the patient to do for himself in that time. That would be called short therapy in the energy healing biz. Occasionally, if I see that a patient just wants me to balance him out every week but is unwilling to put in the time to learn how to help himself, I won't take on the case.

An Ounce of Prevention

In ancient China, the doctor was paid to keep you healthy preventively. If you got sick, you stopped paying him! Whether we're talking about conventional medicine or energy healing, preventative health is the best of all worlds.

Another major factor to consider is which systems are particularly good for certain kinds of illnesses or conditions. Sometimes, the situation won't call for a treatment-oriented intervention, but rather some classes in one of the systems allied with energy healing.

For example, your lower-back stiffness, low energy, and shoulder tension might respond beautifully to a basic class in hatha yoga or t'ai chi. You might learn how to isolate muscle groups and relax them, how to build tone, some basic centering techniques that will help you relax, and, most important, how to incorporate basic breathing techniques into movement.

This approach may be one of the best forms of energy healing for you at first.

It's pretty common for heart patients in China to be sent to a t'ai chi class. Your muscles will gain flexibility, tone, and strength and, because you're undertaking an ongoing exercise regimen, the long-term results will be greater.

Some people, especially younger ones, prefer an exercise system that's a little more physical than the slow-moving t'ai chi. In China, many undertake training in wu shu, which literally means martial arts and usually refers to the more vigorous styles: sword-play, kung fu, or shaolin animal styles of movement like crane, tiger, mantis, monkey, and snake. You could even study panda-style kung fu, but be sure to go easy on the dumplings!

Updating the Ancient

In the beginning of the twentieth century, the Chinese government banned many of the ancient martial arts as dangerous. The Cultural Revolution brought back many of them as daily exercises in schools and community centers, much like calisthenics in the West. The systems were purged of many of their spiritual aspects, as well as some of the more lethal techniques, becoming more acrobatic and stylized—much better than having a threatening, underground system.

Certain extreme techniques, such as yoga's headstand, are easier to learn than you might imagine and offer tremendous health benefits. Naturally, they must be prepared for physically, taught carefully, and done gradually. If the headstand is taught badly, or practiced incorrectly, it can be hazardous to your health. Don't try to learn it from a book; it would be better/smarter/healthier not to do it at all than to do it incorrectly. And if you think I'm going to tell you to check with your doctor to confirm that the headstand is okay for your health condition, you're right. Check it out.

But here's another thought: try to find a doctor who's familiar with the techniques (how they work, what they do for you health-wise, what the potential dangers might be, and so on). Many conventional doctors are trained more in disease than in wellness. For them, if you're symptom-free, you're healthy. It would be difficult for them to render an unbiased decision about something about which they have little training or interest. That's why it's important to take time in choosing doctors as well as energy healers.

Here's another important question to ask yourself: Is your particular health issue chronic or acute? And does a particular school of healing address it?

No bona fide healer wants to turn away a patient in need without trying to help, but healers and healing systems have certain areas of illness in which they specialize or with which they have more consistent success.

When I began doing energy healing, I had the most success in three areas.

The first was with allergies and asthma. A very large percentage of the asthma patients I worked with eliminated the use of inhalers entirely, and over 70 percent drastically cut down on or eliminated the need for oral medication.

I also had much success in problems with the female reproductive system, including fibroids, amenorrhea, dysmenorrhea, and infertility. I often joke how many babies have been born thanks to my participation. (I know how bad that sounds!)

And last, I had success with patients with long-term chronic pain that had no physiological basis.

One particular case comes to mind that encompassed two of those categories. A woman brought a friend, a professional puppeteer who had been suffering with elbow pain for eight years, to see me. After literally 30 seconds of RB, his pain disappeared. It was one of those instances where an old energy scar had persisted after the body had healed. If a healer can target that blockage, the result is often instantaneous, as it was in this case. The woman who had brought him remarked jokingly, "So why can't you do that for my asthma?" When I told her I didn't know she even had asthma, she set up an appointment with me for the next day.

My friend had been suffering with asthma for over 20 years, dealing with it with medication. She also was using an inhaler up to 10 times a day. After our first energy balancing, she felt so good that after a day or two of not needing the inhaler at all, she decided to stop all medication cold turkey; her husband was an MD who could monitor her carefully.

Never make the choice of stopping physician-prescribed medication without your doctor's involvement. Some medications allow that; others require that you be weaned off slowly and under the watchful eye of a physician.

The last time I saw her, five years later, she told me she'd never gone back on the medication. She also said she rarely had even the slightest asthmatic symptoms and when she did, usually at times of great stress, she realized that she hadn't been doing her RB and breathing every day, as she was taught. As soon as she began again, the minor problems disappeared. Now she doesn't miss a day.

How do you know whether a particular healing school has a good success record with a particular complaint? Ask the healer, as well as people who have gone through the treatment. These days, you can find online chat rooms that enable you to be in touch with people who have tried different modalities and had success or failure with a particular health issue. But be careful—I wouldn't base any important decisions on what a stranger who may or may not be reliable says in a chat room.

Separating the Real Healers from the Fakes

There are charlatans who will pretend to be something they're not for a fast buck in every field. To make matters worse, the training systems for so many things in our society are a mad race to collect diplomas and certificates touting expertise far too prematurely. Even a diploma can be forged. I see stories in the media all the time about "doctors" who've never seen the inside of a medical school who've prescribed drugs to unsuspecting patients. In the case of conventional medicine, this can be fatal.

With energy healing, things are a little murkier. There are people who have had a few successes with the laying on of hands or prayer and decided to declare themselves healers. They probably won't do any damage and might even do some good. But by giving the wrong advice, they could also rob patients of critical time with a physician who might have treated the problem easily and with no harm. By totally missing the cause of the problem, they might misdirect someone into believing one thing when the problem is something else entirely.

I personally prefer an old-school approach to training in energy healing, the master/apprentice method. You study with a recognized master of the art until he or she feels you're ready to go out and practice on your own. Unfortunately, that approach isn't always possible anymore; there are too many students and too few masters. At the very least, look for a school that has a strong mentoring system with a master at the helm. This provides some degree of quality control.

An Old-School Approach

The days of the master/apprentice approach are mostly gone. Today, both masters and students need to make a living, and that approach can take a long time even in the best of circumstances. But the prevalent form of training we're seeing nowadays isn't the best answer, either: a 30-hour course followed by a certificate that says you're ready to practice as an expert. I may be old-fashioned, but I try to reserve words like expert and master for something a little more thorough and enduring.

The legendary Shaolin Temple in China is well known for being the birthplace of animal-style martial arts. It may surprise you, however, to know that Shaolin monks were as skilled at healing as they were in fighting, spending 3 of their 10 years of training focused on the healing arts. Admittance into the school was no easy task. According to legend, every winter parents would bring their children to stand barefoot in the snow in a deep horse stance for hours to show their resolution to become students. The master, inside and unseen, would watch carefully for any defect in their character, like complaining, gossiping, or cheating. Those unsuitable candidates were sent home, while a few finalists were invited inside for tea. The master served the tea and told them to drink. If they did, they were eliminated as well; they showed lack of courtesy and respect by not letting the master drink first, even though he'd been the one to tell them to drink. Old school ….

The problem is the smorgasbord/full-meal syndrome. I feel more comfortable with someone who isn't a jack-of-all-trades but rather a master of one. The more certificates I see on the wall or listed on the business card of a healer, the more wary I am. Don't get me wrong: I'm all for the healer undertaking continuing training. What I'm not in favor of is the person who's a collector of systems, who has the most basic training in a lot of different things but hasn't taken the time to perfect any of them.

So how do you spot a less-trained healer or, worse, one who might be a charlatan? Do your homework. Talk to people, and search for information on the internet, remembering to be mindful of the source. Don't be afraid to make an appointment and interview them. See if you get the right vibes during that interview. See if they're forthcoming with answers to your questions. And for heaven's sakes, don't dismiss all your physicians overnight.

A conventional doctor with knowledge—or at least an interest—in energy healing could be your best asset. She may be able to recommend the best modality for your situation. More often, you might hear the following from your physician: "I don't think it will work, but it won't do any harm so I suppose you can give it a try." Take what you can get!

The Patient's Responsibilities

As a patient in energy healing, you have two major responsibilities, and they both end up being the same thing: do your homework.

The first responsibility of a healing patient is due diligence before getting started. Make sure you're in the hands of the right person. As I've already said, do your homework before you start.

The second responsibility is to do your homework *after* you start. If the healer wants you to undertake a practice of breathing, centering, meditation, or herbs, do it. If he wants you to alter your diet somewhat, or take a homeopathic remedy, do it. You can't do things halfway. Energy healing is holistic, not symptomatic, and a variety of elements may be necessary to effect the healing. Often energy healing isn't just someone doing something to you; it's you, helping yourself.

I can't use the dentist analogy enough. You can go for a cleaning and checkup every four or six months, but you have to do your part, too. Brush and floss and take care of your gums. Dentistry is one of the few medical professions where the doctor routinely teaches the patients what they can do to help themselves preventively.

It's Not a Buffet

In energy healing you can't pick and choose from diets, herbs, and treatments as if you're baking a cake without a recipe, making things up as you go along. If an all-carb diet works for some people and an all-protein one works for others, you can't do a little of each and get the results they got. Each diet is balanced and structured within its own parameters. If you're going to do it, do it; follow the protocol or don't bother starting.

The Cost and Duration of Energy Healing

The subject of money is a sticky one. In a perfect world, healers would serve selflessly all those in need. While that might work in a small village, where the local shaman is revered and supported by all, in the real world that's just a pipe dream.

Healers have to receive compensation for what they do unless they have an independent source of income and choose to work for the common good. Some set up a price scale based on patients' ability to pay. Other healers, who want a more elaborate working space and hire support staff, will have greater overhead. Some have more training than others and have spent a lot more time and money on that education; don't they deserve greater compensation? A few healers get rare support from insurance companies, but that isn't common, except for conventional physicians who've changed their approach to a more holistic one.

In fact the idea of doctors performing acupuncture is somewhat ironic to those of us who've been around energy healing for a while. For years, medical doctors pooh-poohed it, calling it trickery. These days you're more likely to see MDs fighting to make sure no one else is allowed to do acupuncture. It boils down to this: a doctor with 100 hours of training can get an acupuncture license and insurance reimbursement, while a Chinese acupuncturist with a lifetime of training and experience but no medical training can't.

I'm not against compensation to a healer for time and effort. Common sense will suggest what's appropriate for both short- and long-term modalities. It should be fair and not exploitive.

But let me make an important point: in more cosmic terms, a patient has to give something to get something in return. If the healer makes the effort and asks for nothing, there's an imbalance in the equation. The patient may feel indebted to the healer and, possibly, somewhat dependent. That's not a good circumstance for energy healing and can lead to problems, possibly even impeded healing. But the compensation doesn't have to be money. The barter system has worked well throughout history, or a special gift for the healer to show the patient's gratitude.

In today's world, people place value on monetary equivalence. The more something costs, the better it must be. Careers in the business world are made by people whose only job is to determine what the market will bear.

Be careful when you enter the energy healing domain. Be cautious but fair. Healers have to eat, too, you know!

 If your gut tells you that the demands a healer is making are too steep—financial or otherwise—or that something doesn't seem right about the whole setup, you're probably right. Trust your instinct. Be very cautious of anyone who tells you that you must give up your conventional medical doctor. Thank him for his time and tell him you'd like to think about it some more. But if things feel right, and you've done your due diligence beforehand, give it a try.

Expectations During and After an Energy Healing Session

When you go to an energy healer, you should have some information regarding what will take place. That way there are no false expectations that prevent you from getting the most out of your encounter. On the other hand, don't limit yourself to what you know; keep an open mind to what may be some wonderful surprises.

Pain or No Pain

Depending on the type of healing system, things may hurt for a bit. Despite the fact that there are no needles or electric shocks (as in acupuncture or electro-acupuncture, respectively), massage systems are the ones likely to leave the most discomfort, especially in deep tissue work. Keep in mind that the pain you experience during palpation is an indicator that something is out of balance, provided the healer isn't exerting excessive pressure. The unexpected pain you feel at the contact point is your body telling you you've reached the underground energy river of chi. If the pain stops when the healer releases the pressure, you'll know the pain is coming from the teh chi (refer to Chapter 8) and not simply a massage healer pushing too hard and bruising you.

It's not uncommon to have some residual pain and limited tissue bruising, but if you're working with a well-trained healer, that should go away in a day or two, hopefully along with the pain or ailment you came in for.

Obviously, the least painful experiences are the laying-on-of-hands systems, where there might not even be any physical contact at all.

Things Getting Worse, Things Getting Better

Ideally, we're all looking for one of those magical moments when pain simply disappears, as it did for the puppeteer earlier in this chapter. Those moments are wonderful for both the patient and the healer. But here's a more common scenario: you go to an energy healer for shoulder pain, he treats you, but when you go home, the pain is actually worse.

It's important to remember that energy blocks, from a holistic point of view, may be thought of more accurately as energy profiles. They might encompass multiple chakras, meridians, physical or emotional factors, and so forth. It's rarely as simple as a localized energy scar from a bicycle injury that gets blown away in a minute or two.

Because energy healing may accelerate the body's natural healing timetable, the symptomatic pain can sometimes get worse after a session. That kind of worsening, in my experience, doesn't last. It usually fades away in 24–48 hours and, hopefully, takes the original symptom along with it.

Fast or Long-Term Results

There's no way of knowing how long it will take for a symptom to go away, or whether it will come back. If the healer finds the energy block or profile that was the cause of the symptom, a rapid healing will often follow. But if the healer only contacted the energy block of the symptom, not the cause, the pain may diminish for a few minutes but come right back. Energy healing doesn't cover up pain, as medications sometimes do; it either breaks up the causative energy block or it doesn't. Sometimes the pain will diminish more slowly, like a balloon with a pinprick hole in it. It doesn't disappear instantaneously; it seeps away slowly, over a day or two.

If the causative energy block is only partially eliminated, the initial symptom may disappear, with some new symptoms taking its place. And those unveiled symptoms may sometimes be on an emotional level, making them subtler and more difficult to isolate. Remember, a symptom sometimes appears to alert you to another underlying problem. The problem may be obvious, but it can just as easily be hidden. Either way, pay attention to these messages and have them looked at by either a healer or a conventional doctor, or both. Get all the information you can on all levels.

The Effect of Energy Healing on Chronic Problems

From an energy healing point of view, there are two types of chronic problems: those in which the cause of the disease is still there, such as leg pain from a torn cartilage in the knee, and those in which the original cause of the symptoms is gone, but the energy scar remains.

Energy healing is often effective in the latter, if the healer is skillful enough to locate and break up the energy block. In the former, where the body can't heal itself, the pain might be somewhat reduced but won't go away until the problem is fixed. Energy healing can't cover it up. Nor would you want it to, as the pain is a reminder to be careful when you walk and exercise.

Let's say you have a bum knee. If you take a muscle relaxant and pain reliever, you won't feel any pain in your knee. You might even think it's all right to go out and run a marathon. Don't! You can do serious damage as a result. Use moderation and common sense: you've masked some pain and you've relaxed some muscles. Now give nature a chance to heal the body.

In cases where energy healing can't eliminate the ailment, it can often speed up the natural healing of the body. Years ago a piano teacher and professor at the North Carolina School of the Arts had broken his arm skiing. He had a major concert in six weeks, but the cast wasn't coming off for a week after that. He'd heard wonderful stories about my work with a number of the Winston-Salem symphony solo instrumentalists and wanted to know if there was anything I could do for him.

I worked on him once a week for three weeks, balancing his energy and spending a little extra time focusing on the point of his break. When he went in for his three-week check-up, the doctor took an X-ray and, based on the X-ray alone, thought the pianist was there for the *six-week* check-up. Not only that, but he said that the bone was healing a little ahead of schedule and had gone through seven weeks of healing and the cast could come off that day. When the pianist corrected him, explaining that it had only been three weeks since the break, the doctor was perplexed. How could the teacher possibly have gone through seven weeks of healing in only three weeks?

The concert went on as scheduled three weeks later, with plenty of time for him to get his arms and hands back in shape.

Years ago, the Russians did research in speeding up the healing of bones by using electrical fields or magnets. This was dismissed as nonsense for a long time. Now, it's not uncommon to have electrical wires placed inside a cast and have electrical fields bathe the broken bone. Healers have been using humanly generated E.L.F. fields for centuries to accomplish the same thing.

While some extraordinary cases of accelerated healing or even repairing torn cartilage have been known to occur, this is beyond the scope of most healers. They can try to get the energy matrix to send a message to the DNA to tell the cartilage to fix itself, but you're probably better off seeking arthroscopic surgery.

Essential Takeaways

- Do your homework before choosing an energy healer.
- When interviewing a healer, trust your instincts; they're usually right.
- Don't give up your medical doctor; a combination of conventional medicine and energy healing is usually the best way to go.
- Once you've chosen a healer, follow his or her instructions. These systems are self-contained and self-balanced; don't pick and choose within the system.

chapter 19

Questions to Ask About Becoming an Energy Healer

Choosing an energy healing modality

Preparing for interviews

Answers to some frequently asked questions

You may have had successful energy healing for a problem of your own. You may have been excited by what you've read in this or other books. You may have always had the feeling that energy healing was something you wanted to learn to do. You may have even had an experience where you laid your hands on someone's injury and the person felt better. You want to be a healer. Here are some things to consider next.

Getting Started: Your Due Diligence

As you read through some of the earlier chapters and became familiar with different modalities, you've undoubtedly had thoughts like "I'll never put needles in anyone!" or "I could learn to do laying on of hands," or "I like crystals; maybe I could get into energy healing that way."

If massage is your thing, begin your due diligence by investigating schools in your area that teach massage.

Search the internet to see what the various schools say. Look for chat rooms of people who've gone there. Check the Better Business Bureau to make sure the school's a legitimate institution with a proven track record and no indications of problems.

You may have to go out of town to find a good school; does your current job or family situation allow for that? I've known lots of teachers who are off in the summer months and do extensive training then. It may take longer to complete the training that way, but they'll get there eventually. A teacher once told me that you don't have to hurry if you're going the right way!

Once you have a list of potential schools, go for a visit. Rather than just ask a lot of questions, I like to experience the healing method for myself; it's the best way to get a feel for the approach. Don't think too much during the session. Just be passive and experience it and save the analysis for later. You have only one real question when it's over: is this something you'd feel comfortable and inspired to learn and practice?

When touring a potential school of healing, follow your gut. If something rubs you the wrong way, thank them for their time and leave. Don't get into a debate; if their school isn't for you, it's not for you.

Even before your first visit to a school, you should ask yourself what kind of healer you want to be. The great Lebanese-American philosopher and poet Kahlil Gibran taught this:

> The teacher who is indeed wise does not bid you to
> enter the house of his wisdom but rather leads you to
> the threshold of your mind.

Learning in this area is a lifetime process that never ends. Keep at it. The more training you have, the better you'll be prepared to serve. As a white belt, I asked Grand Master Sober what a master was. He said, "With effort, you can learn and be expert at many skills; but your goal should be to master only one: *yourself!*" Continuing to grow and mastering the self allows you the opportunity to help others. Don't take a one-month course and decide you know enough to hang up a shingle. Noah Ben Shea, the philosopher who wrote *Jacob the Baker* and other books, said, "What grows, never grows old." Be patient.

Choosing a System: Ask the Right Questions

When you visit a potential school, talk to the director. Ask if it would be all right to speak with some of the students (both beginner and advanced) who have gone through the training. Ask some of the questions outlined in this section. In addition to giving you a good sense of the program, it will demonstrate to the teacher/director that you're serious about this training and not a dabbler.

What is the essence of your system? The first thing you should know is which category of modality is utilized (laying on of hands, gentle or deep-tissue massage, needles, crystals, etc.). Be sure this is an approach you're comfortable with before you go any further. It's also a good idea to find out what sort of problems the system has the most success with.

Can anyone learn to practice the system? You want to know right away if this is a course for beginners or if there are prerequisites you must take before entering the program, such as anatomy or physiology. If those things are part of the curriculum, you'll need to know about it.

Assuming I complete the training, what kind of certification does your school offer? Depending on where you live, you might need a state license to be able to "touch" a patient or client. Many schools have a certification prep course.

How long is the training program for practitioners? That will depend on how technical the system is. If you're interested in acupuncture, homeopathy, or other systems in which you must memorize properties of herbs, meridians, or others points, that will take a while. On the other hand, some of the more intuitive modalities—laying on of hands, for example—can be learned more quickly.

How do you determine whether I'm right for your school? This is a question that's more appropriate for a private teacher than a school. Don't forget, while you're interviewing a teacher, that person is also interviewing you! She may not want to commit a lot of time to someone she doesn't consider serious, or someone who doesn't possess some natural gift for energy healing. If that's the case, how does she make that determination? Is it through psychic intuition, or is there some kind of test you have to take to see if you're qualified?

Be cautious with teachers who accept you psychically for an expensive training program. It could be authentic, but it could also be a marketing strategy for attracting high-paying students. Don't let flattery get the better of you.

Does your system encourage the healer to teach students how to sustain results on their own? Throughout this book, we've talked about the importance of teaching healing patients how to balance themselves, a key component to holistic medicine. But what if you're not a teacher? Does that mean you can't be a healer? Absolutely not! There are many modalities that don't focus as much on teaching the patient how to sustain the results. Make sure you know whether the school you're interested in teaches you to just work on the patients, or if the healing encounter includes teaching the patient.

Is there a specific diagnostic approach in your system, or is it based on the patient's history? In some modalities, the patient tells the healer what the problem is and he begins working on it. In other systems—t'ai chi healing, for example—the healer may take readings of the Chinese pulses, look at the tongue or face, or ask if certain points are tender to the touch. Other systems of electro-acupuncture may take readings with a machine to determine imbalances.

If you prefer using machines for diagnosis, the Nakatani Ryodoraku machine takes readings (in the range of 1–100 millivolts) from test points on the fingers and toes, called seiketsu points, and thereby determines which meridians are out of balance. The machine can be hooked up to a computer so results can be generated quickly, both before and after treatment. An expert pulse-taker will do just as well, though obviously less objectively.

Is there any supportive research on your particular system? Not every school that teaches energy healing has been involved in research. That's okay; anecdotal success stories may be enough for you. But if you want to see supportive research, ask if there's any available within that school. A nurse, for example, might be interested in some of the research that's been done in Therapeutic Touch; this modality, as explained in Chapter 7, was founded by a nurse, Delores Krieger, PhD. Someone with a nursing background might even want to participate in any ongoing research.

Is the system focused only on physical ailments, or is there an emotional component, too? Many people with backgrounds in psychology, psychiatry, or social work are interested in the psycho-emotional arena of energy healing. They'll want to know whether a particular school of healing deals with that. In t'ai chi healing, energy profiles (or syndromes, as they're sometimes called), not symptoms, are the basis of treatment. These profiles encompass yin-yang and five-element theory, which by their very nature incorporate emotional factors into their diagnosis and treatment.

When t'ai chi healing says that anger is related to the liver and gall bladder meridians and fear to the kidney and urinary bladder meridians, it should be clear that these emotions may not be understood in exactly the same way as Western medicine or psychology understands them. If you come from that Western model, keep an open mind to new ways of looking at things.

Is there a religious component to your system? If so, do I have to be of that faith or believe in its tenets to practice it? Some healing systems have a strong religious component, which can lead to uncomfortable situations if you're of a different faith. Some yoga schools involve puja, religious ceremonies with offerings, chanting, and the naming of Indian gods. That might make some people uncomfortable. This is a personal question you should ask yourself, but as a rule of thumb, if a foreign language is used in healing, make sure you know what you're saying and that it doesn't bother you in any way.

These questions can help prepare you before you go in for an interview. You don't need to ask every one of them, but try to think through the areas that are important to you beforehand, and don't be shy about getting answers. When people come to talk with me, I appreciate it when they're prepared with questions. I enjoy the dialogue.

Potential Risks: From Energy Weakness to Karma

There are many misconceptions about energy healing. I think it's important for every aspiring healer to be familiar with some of the more common of them so they know how to respond.

If I engage in energy healing, will I feel weak or drained afterward? No, not if you do it the right way. When you're grounded, you've plugged in to the earth's 2-billion-volt electrical potential and have access to plenty of energy, provided you're on the correct 8 hz wavelength. It's similar to using a laptop computer: if it's plugged into the wall, it doesn't run down. If it's only on battery power, it does. *Your* energy isn't what's doing the work in healing; it's your energy matrix phase-locked with the earth. Many healers say that they feel more energized after a long healing session, as opposed to feeling drained.

If I engage in energy healing, will I take on the disease of my patient? This can be an issue but is easily remedied with proper training and preparation. If you're rooted, and you wash your hands before and after each session, you'll be fine. In this case, the roots are used not for the purpose of drawing the energy in, but as a lightning rod to dissipate the negative energy plaque you might come in contact with during the course of the healing.

I knew a woman who did wonderful healing work with crystals. She always had a few hanging around her neck in a small velvet pouch. Normally, when she finished a healing session, she put the crystal in fresh earth or sunlight to cleanse it.

Once, when she was still new to energy healing, she was asked to help a fellow healer with a pneumonia patient. She took one of her clear quartz crystals from her little velvet pouch to use. After drawing off a lot of negative energy from the patient, the crystal literally turned cloudy. But in this case she had a long three-hour ride home in a car, so she put the crystal back in the pouch. She sat dozing quietly in the back seat, with the cloudy crystal hanging around her neck, pressing against her chest.

Later that night she began to show severe pneumonia symptoms. Her doctor checked her out for standard diagnostic markers for pneumonia but didn't find any. Realizing what had happened, she removed the crystal from the bag, cleaned it, and then had a friend help her cleanse her energy matrix. In less than an hour, the symptoms were gone.

It is of the utmost importance to take simple precautions like being grounded and washing hands before and after any healing session. I don't mean to sound like a broken record, but I want your experience in receiving or giving energy healing to be safe for you.

Will I take on the karma of someone I work on who shouldn't be healed? This is one of the questions I'm asked quite often, but I find it reveals a misunderstanding of what karma actually is. Karma refers to the ledger of good and bad actions a soul can take in his or her life. It doesn't mean fate. You make choices in life, and the product of those choices and actions is your karma. It's not transferable; a person is responsible for his or her own actions.

Remember the two lines from the mantra in Chapter 12?

> Each day, take responsibility for your physical performance; each day, take responsibility for your mental performance.

That's all about karma. You live with the consequences of your choices and actions. Moreover, when all the plusses and minuses cancel each other out at the end of your life, what's left—both positive and negative—is what you take into your next life. It's yours; you can neither give it to someone else nor escape it.

More important, if your intention in the healing encounter was to channel positive energy to help the patient, and for some cosmic reason this person's destiny was not to be cured or healed, you take on no debt. You tried, and you earn the positive energy of that choice and action, nothing else. Think of it like a banker trying to help someone refinance his home loan. If the banker can't make the numbers work, he's not suddenly responsible for the customer's mortgage!

FAQs About Energy Healing

We've gone over questions you may want to ask yourself before choosing a modality and questions to ask of a potential teacher or learning institution. There are a few others I feel every healer should be prepared for.

Do I have to have a special gift to be an energy healer? It doesn't hurt, but it isn't necessary. I've been fortunate to work with and train some naturally gifted healers in my life, Dr. Andrew Chernick, D.Ac., among them. He's now the head master-teacher of RB and EnerGenesis in Israel. He trains healers and sees patients and has a wondrous healing gift. You may remember the story I told in Chapter 10 about how he inadvertently discovered his own version of remote healing when he crossed his legs over his wife's.

Andrew was with me at almost every stage of RB and EnerGenesis as it developed over the years, and many of its innovations are attributable to his suggestions, challenges, and applications.

I am equally proud of another gifted healer, Dr. Harvey Grossbard, OMD. Harvey has been a Professor of Oriental Medicine at a number of professional schools in Florida, California, and Israel and is a top-notch acupuncturist, herbalist, and homeopath, with highly developed energy skills.

The final word, however, is that you don't need to have some inborn gift to heal. We all have the potential to become a superb energy healer. It takes character, patience, perseverance, and time.

With so many people around who need energy healing, why don't healers offer themselves to others more frequently? There's a prime directive in the world of energy healing (please forgive yet another *Star Trek* reference): patients need to ask for energy healing. That prepares them to be open and ready to receive the healing, whether they know it or not. Every bona fide healer I've ever met felt the same way, some of them pretty well known in the field. It seems to be accepted universally.

So what do you do if you encounter someone you believe you can help but she hasn't asked you for assistance? You can bring up the subject or sway the conversation to related topics. Just let her be the one to ask and open the door.

I admit that, in a world where so many people have started hanging up shingles in various modalities of energy healing, not as many healers hold to this practice. Nevertheless, I've found it to be sound.

I've heard that some healers use drugs or herbs to get into a healing state. Is that necessary? This is a difficult question to answer. For centuries, even millennia, shamans the world over have used tobacco, mushrooms, and other sacred plants to induce a readiness to achieve higher states of consciousness and participate in energy healing. In his first book, *The Sacred Mushroom*, Dr. Puharich documented civilizations that have revered *Amanita muscaria* and its mystical, mind-expanding properties for thousands of years. In *Beyond Telepathy*, he shared his research among shamans and yogis and attempted to offer his early thoughts on the science behind remote viewing. The use of hallucinogenic substances wasn't uncommon in those cultures to aid in expanding one's consciousness. These cultures and traditions, though, have deep histories. Without the right preparation, great dangers exist.

> **stay Grounded** — Just a few years ago, on a walk through a sacred woods in Arizona, a Native American–trained shaman showed me a plant that, when properly prepared, induced a very deep trance. When improperly prepared though, he told me, it was fatal. It took years before his teachers would trust him with its preparation. Don't fool around with this stuff.

Back in the 1970s, I met a healer with amazing gifts. When he healed, he could literally see inside the patient. He could describe plaque inside an artery in detail, only to have it confirmed with conventional diagnostic technology. His accuracy was uncanny. His hands turned beet red when he worked and his energy was palpable to those who sat nearby. The only problem was that he believed he only could do this under the influence of illegal substances. Several greater authorities, including Puharich, believed he was using them as a crutch and could have done as well without it.

Clearly, using something that's illegal isn't an acceptable choice. But I think it goes beyond that. Those who use drugs do so to achieve triaspheric divergence, enabling the inner eye of imagination to expand, to attach their energy matrix to the WEB, and see things most regular folks can't.

But there are many other cultures in which these substances aren't used, and the same states of mind are achieved through breathing and meditation. In fact, the teachers in those cultures are against introducing any type of outside agent or substance into the body.

I have no doubt that ancient systems safely mastered the preparation and use of these substances. I wouldn't presume to judge a particular culture's practices, especially one that has millennia of success behind it. Nevertheless, my personal belief is that if healing can be done without the use of outside substances, that's preferable.

You said that to become a healer requires character, patience, perseverance, and time. What do you mean by time?

Healing isn't just about technique; it's about people. It's about building a world community that's in balance and harmony. It's about sharing light and sweetening the world. It's easy to get caught up in the technique and craft of energy healing, whatever modality you choose, and forget why you got into the world in the first place. As a beautiful Zen saying goes, "When pointing at the moon, don't confuse the finger with the moon."

The *Sufis* have a story about time and pomegranates. Once upon a time, a young man went to a revered Sufi teacher because he wanted to become an apprentice and learn the Sufi methods and secrets. The teacher was impressed with his sincerity and accepted him as a student.

Finding Meaning

Sufism is the mystical branch of Islam, much as Kabbalah is the mystical branch of Judaism. Some of its adherents maintain that Sufism is a universal truth, beyond silence, the distillation of all great truths. The Sufi has gone beyond the maya (illusion) and karma of the world and is centered only in God.

One day, an old man came to the home of the Sufi seeking healing. The teacher, seeing the man from the distance, remarked to the apprentice that he would need pomegranates to be healed. When the man approached, he explained the sad situation that had led to his illness and asked for help. After listening to the whole story, the Sufi sat in meditation for several moments. Then he said, "I believe that your life force is in a state of imbalance. You will need certain energies to set it right. You will need the color of red to excite the life force; you will need something tart as an opposite to stimulate a sweetness that is needed within you, and you will need something filled with the seeds of new life to stimulate growth. Ah, I have it! The perfect thing! Eat three pomegranates a day for a week and you will be healed."

The grateful patient left. A week later, he returned, completely healthy. With tears in his eyes, he thanked the Sufi and brought him baskets of fruits and sweets as a tribute to his wisdom.

The next day, a second man approached from the distance. The Sufi remarked that this patient also needed pomegranates. The student said, "Master, now that you have done the work and diagnosed him, may I be the one to deliver the treatment?" The teacher agreed.

As the man came near, the student stood up and said, "I know what you need! You need to eat three pomegranates a day for a week!" The man, outraged, yelled at him. "I have come all this way and I haven't even told you what is wrong, and you spout this nonsense about pomegranates! Bah!" In a rage he turned and walked away.

The student was perplexed.

> "I don't understand, Master. You said he needed pomegranates and I told him so. Why did he become angry and leave?"
>
> "Ah, my young apprentice, you still have much to learn. That's not all the patient needed. He needed pomegranates and *time*."

The moral of the story: you're not just healing meridians and chakras; you're privileged to be helping to heal people. It requires character, patience, perseverance, and above all else, time.

Essential Takeaways

- If you want to be a healer, experience the system as a patient first. That will tell you whether or not you want to pursue training in that modality.
- Do your homework about an energy healing system before you go in for an interview.

- Be prepared with a list of questions about things you want to know from the healer or director of the school.
- As you listen to the answers, read between the lines about everything—from karma to cost—to get a better sense of the school's true philosophy.
- Listen to your gut to see whether a particular form of energy healing is the right match for you.
- Never use illegal substances to enhance your healing ability, regardless of whether or not they work.

chapter 20

Energy Healing Cases

Cases that disappoint and surprise

Learning from "impossible" cases

On death, dying, and energy healing

The well-accepted idea that teachers learn as much from their students as the students learn from the teachers couldn't be any truer than it is in the world of energy healing. So many of the lessons I've learned over the decades have come from cases I've been part of. Sometimes the lessons came from the patient and sometimes they came in retrospect from the case as a whole. I'd like to share some of those lessons with you in this chapter.

The Most Disappointing Energy Healing Cases

The first ones that come to mind are people I was close to who had terminal illnesses whom I was unable to help. Some asked for healing, some didn't. The notion in conventional medicine is that you shouldn't treat family and relatives. That's completely understandable but not necessarily true in energy healing. There are many people close to me who I've been able to help over the years. In one case where the patient was a relative, a fibroid tumor the size of an orange disappeared in a matter of days. That blew everyone's minds, especially my relative's doctor!

But sometimes the mindset of a person doesn't allow him to ask for help. He may have personal baggage that prevents him from asking a family member for help. It's sad, but that's the way it is. Sometimes you think you can help but aren't given the opportunity. I won't do a formal healing unless I've been asked. I have no problem sending out prayers for people, but I won't tread around someone's energy matrix without an invitation.

Another kind of disappointment comes when close friends extend the invitation, but for whatever cosmic reason it just isn't enough. In some cases, I wasn't able to tune in to their energy matrix, or I didn't have the ability needed to channel enough energy to produce the needed change.

I can't say that my attempts didn't provide any healing for the individual, even if they didn't bring the cure we were hoping for. Maybe the effort bought them some extra time to come to peace with what was happening to them. Nevertheless, it still hurts a bit when you can't help one person (especially someone close to you) with the same problem you were successful with in another case. You do what you can, you stay as optimistic as you can, and trust that the universe is unfolding as it should be.

One of my favorite poems is known as the Desiderata, written by Max Ehrmann (1872–1945). The final verse reads: You are a child of the universe, no less than the trees or the stars; you have a right to be here. And, whether or not it is clear to you, no doubt the universe is unfolding as it should.

Sometimes you have the ability to help, but the patient isn't ready to receive. Remember, there are radio waves all around us, but you can't hear anything unless you turn on your radio. We have free will and can choose, consciously or unconsciously, whether we want to receive healing energy. Two cases come to mind where the patients could see the possibilities of energy healing and still decided it wasn't for them for reasons I couldn't comprehend.

The first was a woman with breast cancer, discovered at an early-enough stage that it seemed beatable. She came to me for additional energy healing, to hedge her bets, I guess. At the first session her energy profile showed a good response. I taught her some breathing, rooting, and basic RB that had to do with her immune system and the breast area, to keep the healing energy moving. I commented that she might have to trim her thumbnails a bit, because to do RB with long, beautifully cared-for nails like hers would have been difficult.

When she came back the next week, the improvement in the energy matrix had held, and she felt a lot better. She said she couldn't do the RB, however, because of her long nails (as if we hadn't discussed it at the first session). We talked about trimming them again, and she assured me she would. She was so happy with the results so far; she said she felt more energized and healthier than she had in a long time.

When she arrived for the third session, nails intact, I saw the writing on the wall: she'd never had any intention of trimming her well-manicured thumbs. Apparently keeping her extremely long thumbnails won out over the ability to work on her energy matrix. Maybe it's just me, but this was hard to understand. After all, the nails would grow back. She could have used artificial nails that matched her real ones for a short time. I'm not sure what happened to her; I wished her well and told her to keep practicing what she'd learned.

If that case surprises you, this one will blow your mind. A 72-year-old nurse, who had been a heavy smoker for years and had emphysema, came to see me. Now on oxygen regularly, she wanted to know if I could help her breathing. In the course of my taking a history, she told me about her digestion and daily eliminations. She had been using enemas daily for 69 years! She told me she hadn't had a normal bowel movement without an enema for 50 years and used two or three enemas every day. She wasn't constipated; the enemas did the job.

During that first session, I worked on her whole energy matrix and taught her some basic breathing and how to palpate the RB everyday areas, which would take a total of about 10 minutes a day. She was very positive and optimistic.

The next morning she called me, elated. She'd had three normal bowel movements the day before without an enema. She couldn't remember the last time that had happened. I told her to keep up the RB, which had apparently energized her colon, and looked forward to seeing her the next week. At the second session, she told me that she had "normalized" to one bowel movement a day and hadn't used an enema since. And her breathing had improved so that she was now able to do without the oxygen for a few hours at a time, especially while she worked in the kitchen. That was something she loved to do, but she'd had to cut back on because of the oxygen.

The night before the next session, she called to cancel. She wanted to stop our work together and when I asked her why, she said, "The self-massage is too much work for me. It's easier for me to take the enemas, so I've started doing them again. But I'm very happy about the improvement in the breathing, and thanks for all you've done." I got off the phone in a daze. To each her own, I guess … but that one left me floored.

I can hear DeVries's voice in my head: "Don't expect anything positive from human nature and you won't be disappointed. And then, when it happens, be pleasantly surprised!"

There are times when the difference between life and death for someone can be determined by simple words. Nothing brought that closer to home for me than the case in recent months of a friend who "graduated" with a severe brain tumor (graduation is how my late teacher Greta referred to death). According to his doctors, he should have had less than a year to live. I had the opportunity to work both locally and by remote healing with him. He seemed to be doing pretty well for quite some time, with occasional ups and downs and, in fact, lasted two and a half years. For most of that, you wouldn't have known he was ill at all. He was a loving man with a great sense of humor and a close-knit family. He was also a fighter, and he fought hard for the life and family he loved.

The last time I treated him, it felt as if he was no longer open to receiving the energy I was sending him. It was almost like pouring water through a sieve. And he had always been such a fighter! Disappointed, I asked his wife about it. She told me that he had been doing really well until a physical therapist he was working with remarked thoughtlessly one day, "You know, you'll never beat this cancer. It kills everyone." For some reason, he was in a weakened state of mind that day, and his emotional resistance was low; the remark got through his normal defensive persona of optimism. It broke him. He lost hope and the ability to fight. He began a steady decline from that day forward, which led to his death.

Words Have Power

When you work as a healer, it's not just the energy you send with your hands; ugly words make ugly water crystals. Be conscious of what you say. Words can seriously affect your energy flow. Use them with care or not at all. My grandmother was right: if you have nothing nice to say, don't say anything at all!

Each of the cases taught me lessons about human nature. We all have our own paradigms and priorities, and sometimes we have to be willing to yield our own sense of what is right or sensible to another person's choices.

The Most Gratifying Energy Healing Cases

Fortunately, there are more positive cases than negative ones. The lessons here are more gratifying and often joyful. Let's look at a few of them.

The Surprising Cases

I love the cases that have a positive healing result and an additional surprise as well. A 70-year-old woman came to see me with severe hip pain she'd had for several months. She walked with a limp but told me she'd had it since she was a teenager and that it was unrelated to the recent pain. When I asked her to point to the focal point of the pain, she took my hand and pressed it against a specific spot on her hip.

There was a golf-ball-size mass there. When I asked about it, she said she'd had it all her life and that doctors had told her it was benign. The mass had been there for so long, she couldn't remember when she'd first noticed it and it wasn't the cause of the pain. I worked on the related RB points, focused some additional energy on the painful spot, and then asked her to walk across the room again.

The pain was gone! Not only that, the limp she'd had for most of her life was gone, too. On a whim, I asked her to check the mass to see if it had changed. She got a strange look on her face. She couldn't find it. It had been there for over 50 years and it was suddenly gone. The woman had come to see me to help get rid of some pain and got a double surprise: a lifelong limp and mass disappeared as well.

When "miracle" events take place, don't let them go to your head. Keep the ego out of it. You're an instrument of a much larger symphony; enjoy the moment and move on.

Cases That Leave Clear Evidence

Without exaggeration, the case I'm about to describe changed my life more than any other I've ever worked on. The patient was none other than Dr. Andrija Puharich. For years, he'd suffered from recurring bouts of shingles, which is a herpes zoster virus, varicella type, like chicken pox in adults. It is a very uncomfortable disease that can show up as a painful rash anywhere on the body as a ribbon or cluster of lesions. Even after they disappear (in anywhere from two weeks to a month) the ongoing pain, known as post-herpetic neuralgia, can last several months or more.

Up until 1984, when the events I'm about to describe occurred, I thought of myself as a kind of technician-healer. I was pretty good at the massage technique that evolved into RB. I had been able to alleviate pain, help asthma, allergies, a number of female reproductive problems, and chronic pain. But all of this was subjective. There wasn't any physical evidence of an objective cause-and-effect result from the healing work I did.

Having Dr. Puharich for a patient meant that he could explain things about the disease that other patients couldn't. He explained the internal workings of shingles, in addition to the skin lesions. Formations appear in the blood, which Dr. Puharich described as a bag full of bagels all stuck together. When I saw the photographed blood cells, I immediately saw that his not-so-elegant analogy was accurate. Blood cells normally float through the circulatory system, repelling each other like magnets because of their negative surface charge. But when blood cells get tangled up with positively charged antibodies, they begin to clump together. These clumps are called rouleaux formations, French for rolls. This clumping impedes the transfer of oxygen from the blood cells.

Dr. Puharich had just had a new outbreak of lesions the day before I arrived at his home. He asked if I would work on him, adding that it might be interesting to turn it into an experiment. He would shoot some slides of living blood cells in his lab in the basement, see if the rouleaux formations were present, and then proceed to monitor them every day or two to see if any improvements in the blood showed up faster than his usual two-to-three-month timetable. When the acute flare-up ended, which might be in as few as several weeks, the condition of rouleaux formations in the blood lasted two or three weeks after the episode and then cleared up.

I had no expectations about what might occur. My only thought was to root my energy matrix, log on to the WEB, phase-lock with Puharich's energy matrix, and alleviate his discomfort.

Deeper Connections In energy healing, once you start to work, it's best not to focus on your expectations, which is obviously to heal the patient. Just be open to whatever happens. When you work, "just say Y.E.S.": Yield the ego to the higher energy of the WEB, Energize your energy matrix to as high a level as possible, and Share whatever flows through you.

First he photographed some blood samples; then we did the healing. Shortly after we finished, he went back down to the lab to shoot the first set of post-healing pictures of the blood cells. But he didn't come back up. After about half an hour, I went down to find him. He was sitting at the monitor, staring at blood cell photographs. The blood was normal.

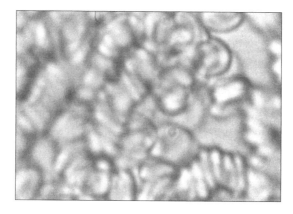

Blood cells before healing.

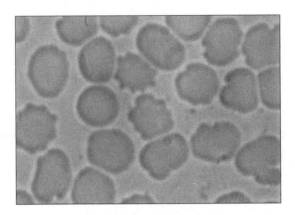

Blood cells after healing.

The rouleaux formations had disappeared! The little rough edges of some of the cells, which he called crenations, were due to the fact that the slide preparation was rather thin, causing the heat of the lamp to dry the blood more quickly than it normally would. The next slide was prepared a little thicker, and the blood looked completely normal; the crenations were gone … in 90 minutes! We were blown away. He had been testing his own blood for years and had never seen anything like this.

This case was significant for the development of RB; it demonstrated chemical change as a direct result of the energy balancing. In this case, RB and EnerGenesis, the energy scanning/treatment components of my system, triggered results in less than 90 minutes. It was also personally significant in that it expanded my own perception of what my capabilities could be as an energy healer.

The Impossible Cases

Working in energy healing, you occasionally witness something that defies explanation.

In the late 1970s my wife had some shredded cartilage in her knee, and it looked like an arthroscopy might be needed to shave it off. She was in a lot of pain and couldn't throw kicks in karate or fold her legs into a lotus posture in yoga classes.

We asked my healing mentor, Greta, if she could do anything to help the pain. Greta began to gently massage the knee. As she continued the massage, she got a look in her eyes that indicated she had entered an unusually deep, altered state. Lillian let her eyes close to feel the warm healing energy from Greta's hands. I closed mine, too, intending to help power-pack Greta by sending her additional energy to accomplish whatever she was doing. After a moment or two, Lillian gasped. We all opened our eyes and looked down.

I can't tell you what actually occurred because to this day I still can't wrap my head around it. It appeared as though Greta's index finger had disappeared, all the way to her second knuckle, inside Lillian's knee! Lillian felt no pain from this; if we weren't all seeing that same thing, I might have thought I was imagining it. Greta slowly withdrew her finger, and we saw some whitish goo on her finger that disappeared within seconds. None of us knew what to make of it. We just sat there, staring at each other, utterly speechless.

As we recovered from the shock, Greta asked Lillian how the knee was. It was still a little weak, but for the first time in months, Lillian pulled her legs in and folded effortlessly into lotus posture. The knee wasn't sore, and all mobility had returned.

Whatever happened that night, which I don't think any of us will ever fully understand, was some form of energy healing from a completely different dimension.

Deeper connections

Whenever I witness something that defies scientific explanation, all I can think of is the famous line from Hamlet: "There are more things in heaven and Earth, Horatio, than are dreamt of in your philosophy."

The more you try to explain some things, the crazier they often sound. Here's my attempt to explain what happened: if we each are an energy matrix inside a WEB, it's theoretically possible that the atoms in Greta's fingers could find their way into the spaces between the atoms of Lillian's knee. That's a pretty tough thing to accept, even as a theoretical possibility, much less as an actual event happening before your eyes.

Let me share one other "impossible" case that's only slightly more down to Earth. It was one of the most dramatic healings I was ever involved in: a woman who had been diagnosed with Glioblastoma, stage 4, a terrible form of brain tumor that grows spiderlike in the brain and is therefore inoperable, with a less than 2 percent chance of survival for two years. The patient was at the end of that time period when we met, and her doctors didn't have much hope of her surviving for longer than a few more weeks.

It seemed as if it was pre-ordained that I work with her: within 24 hours I had received three phone calls—one from Israel, one from Boston, and the last from Miami—each asking if I thought I could help a patient with Glioblastoma. None of the three callers knew each other, but they were calling about the very same person. That was the first sign that something important was going to happen.

Deeper connections

The synchronistic appearance of patients is quite common in the energy healing world. I've experienced it dozens of times, and many healers have told me similar stories.

Whenever there's a type of disease or problem that I seem to be destined to learn about, a whole array of people with that problem show up at my doorstep. It was a little eerie at first, but I came to accept it, and even expect it, after a while.

The woman flew down from Boston. She could barely speak because of the pressure of the tumor on her brain and was unable to make eye contact. In fact, her eyes were mostly closed the first day or two.

I worked with her each day for almost a week. By the end of the week we were having deep conversations, she was laughing freely, and she had no trouble making eye contact. As a matter of fact, her eyes were sparkling when she left at the end of the week and returned to Boston. She seemed to be quite improved, but it was difficult to know if anything was happening internally.

Two weeks later a new brain scan was taken, which was to have been her last by the doctor's timetable. It revealed that the tumor had shrunk by 90 percent! A year later, it was down to 94 percent and her doctors believed that what remained was probably scar tissue. There was no sign of cancer.

Her MD said that in 25 years of working with this type of cancer, he had only occasionally seen it slow down its growth a bit. He had never seen it stop growing entirely, and he had certainly *never* seen it shrink.

The woman died two years later … not of cancer, as it turned out, but from the side effects on her immune system caused by the experimental chemotherapy she had been given, according to her doctor. The cancer hadn't recurred. She was cured *and* healed, made more whole because of the energy healing. She received the gift of time to enable her to get her life together. She called toward the end of her life to thank me for helping her have that time.

Terminal Patients: The Measure of Success or Failure

The final category of energy healing cases is, appropriately, the final point we all reach at some time or another. We all eventually die of something. No human being will escape that, and no amount of energy healing will prevent it.

I learned this lesson firsthand soon after moving to Miami in 1986. After hearing some of the stories I told about energy healing, a karate student asked if I would work on his mother. She had been diagnosed with a very aggressive form of liver cancer. While she vaguely knew who I was, we didn't talk much during the sessions. She came a few times, I tried to scan and balance her energy matrix, and she left. I can't say that anything I did helped much, nor was she in a state of mind to learn a daily routine of breathing or centering. She stopped coming as the disease progressed.

One afternoon, I got a call from her son, who asked me to come to her hospital bedside. She had been comatose for several days and appeared to be at the very end of her life. I sat by her side, praying and sending energy to her energy matrix. Nothing happened, as far as we could tell.

As I left the room and reached the elevators, her son ran into the hallway and called me to come back quickly. By the way he screamed I imagined the worst. I ran up the hall and into the room to find her sitting up in bed, alert. She smiled broadly at me and said, "Hello, Michael!" I was stunned. We've all heard stories about terminal patients experiencing a period of clarity before death, but even the doctors commented on how quickly after the healing she'd come out of the coma. It was as though the energy gave her the jolt she needed to wake up. I was equally surprised, though possibly more so because she greeted me by name; I didn't think she even knew who I was! I gave her a big hug and spoke with her for a few moments. Then I left, allowing the family their private time.

I was told later that she spent about a half hour saying her good-byes to each and every member of the family. She then said she was tired and wanted to rest. She went to sleep and died peacefully.

stay Grounded

When you enter the world of energy healing, you learn to be open to all possibilities. You don't always know what the higher plan is for someone. All you can do is try to stay centered and focused and offer the energy you've been chosen to channel with love and gratitude. Don't try to out-guess the cosmos … you won't win.

This experience wasn't a singular one. Almost the exact same sequence of events happened with my friend/colleague, Dr. Andrew Chernick. As I mentioned in Chapter 10, his father had "seen" me standing at his bedside in Monticello, New York, even though I was engaged in remote healing with him over 100 miles away in New York City.

Five years later, when Andrew's father was in a semi-coma and close to death, Andrew called me in North Carolina and asked if I would do a remote healing from there. As Andrew sat in Monticello on the other end of the phone, I rooted and began to send energy or thoughts of healing to his father through Andrew. In a short time, his father began to stir. Within moments he came out of the semi-coma sufficiently enough to communicate with him, and they had a very meaningful conversation. They had a chance to say good-bye. Andrew's father died later that night.

Even dying takes a certain amount of energy. Think of it like a rocket that needs enough energy thrust to achieve escape velocity through the earth's atmosphere. Sometimes the soul needs energy to escape the body's heavy atmosphere. That's especially true when family members tether the soul to the earth with their love. As a healer, you give your energy with love and compassion and let the soul use that as it needs to, even if you or the family don't agree with or understand its choice.

I feel my participation in this aspect of energy healing is a truly sacred honor and responsibility. To participate in this moment of graduation for the soul is a holy—and holistic—act of love. And while our first objective is to free our patients from disease, helping people become more whole is what energy healing is really all about.

Essential Takeaways

- Don't anticipate what the result of your energy healing will be. The universe is unfolding as it should.
- When the patient is ready, healing can happen. Don't become frustrated if the patient isn't ready; try to be understanding.
- Impossible cases happen from time to time, as do surprise successes. Enjoy the moment and keep the ego out of it.
- Even the death of a patient can be a wondrous act of healing.

Glossary

acupuncture   A complex system of Chinese healing designed to balance the body's energy channels. If the energy is blocked, disease occurs. Treatment can occur through needles, heat, or electricity.

acupressure   A complex system of Chinese healing designed to balance the body's energy channels. If the energy is blocked, disease occurs. Treatment can occur through massage or heat.

Aikido   A Japanese martial art using the force of the attacker to defeat him by redirecting that force from a centered state.

alpha   The brain wave designation for a deep, relaxed state, in the range of 8–14 hz. At low alpha, 8 hz, the mind is highly effective for energy healing, perhaps because this is so close to the natural "heartbeat" of the earth itself.

altered state of consciousness   Refers to the various brain wave patterns we experience, from being fully awake to being asleep.

Ayn-Sof   The two-word phrase that Kabbalists use to refer to God; literally means "no end" or "infinite."

Ayurvedic medicine   A holistic system that strives for balance of body, mind, and spirit through the use of diet, yoga, breathing, meditation, massage, chanting, herbs, etc.

beta   The normal waking-state brain wave of 15–30 hz or cycles per second.

binah   A Hebrew word referring to the divine energy relating to cognitive understanding. This esoteric force is associated with left-brain hemispheric functioning.

biofeedback   Using internal biological systems (e.g., galvanic skin response) or machines to give feedback on a body's state of tension or relaxation.

bpm   Breaths per minute.

Brahm   An Indian term referring to the highest energy possible; the oneness of the universe, the Creator.

Bushido   The highly ethical way of the Japanese Samurai warrior.

caduceus   An ancient symbol that represents the goal of deep meditation: the unification of positive and negative forces (ida and pingala) that heightens the body's spiritual energy potential and frees the serpent (kundalini) force within the energy matrix, leading to higher consciousness. The army medical corps uses the symbol as their logo.

catecholamines   Hormones produced by stress.

chakra   Literally, wheel, the energy matrix's step-down transformers; the energy equivalent of the body's nerve plexuses and endocrine glands combined.

chi   The life-force energy according to the Chinese.

Chi Gung   Energy exercise or energy discipline; comprises whole systems of energy meditation and healing.

cps   Cycles per second, also known as hz (hertz).

Craniosacral Therapy   A system of manual therapy developed by John Upledger, DO, OMM, that seeks to reestablish the flow and pressure of the cerebrospinal fluid in and around the head and spine, leading to enhanced self-healing.

cupping   A way of stimulating acupuncture points by using glass cups and heat.

da'at   The Hebrew word for divine energy related to the deepest form of instantaneous knowing.

dan tien   *See* tan t'ien.

danjeon   *See* tan t'ien.

delta   The brain wave designation for the sleep state (1–3 hz).

divergence   A method of controlling the eyes, ears, or nostrils to induce a light trance. In divergence, the hemispheres of the brain are uncoupled, because each hemisphere is linked to an eye, ear, and nostril.

dosha   In Ayurvedic medicine, the three major metabolic constitutions or body types.

E.L.F.   Extremely Low Frequency magnetic fields in the range of 1–100 hz. Also referred to as scalar waves.

EnerGenesis   A system of energy healing developed by the author to help reestablish balance in the energy matrix.

energy matrix   The author's designation for the body's multi-dimensional energy field. This all-encompassing field's anatomy includes meridians, nadis, chakras, etc. It may be thought of as the equivalent of the aura.

entrainment   The point at which the frequencies of two individuals or objects vibrate together; one frequency entrains the other.

ether   An energy that isn't visible or measurable with current technology, though it's been part of humankind's attempt to understand the life force for millennia.

fight-or-flight response   The physiological mechanism that prepares the body to deal with stressful situations.

fractal   A shape in which each part is a copy of the whole.

Galvanic skin response   One scale used in biofeedback to measure electrical conduction of electricity in the skin, relative to the moisture from perspiration. This scale is used to ascertain the level of stress in the individual.

gung fu   *See* kung fu.

hado   A Japanese term for the life force.

hara   The Japanese term for the body's lower center of gravity; *See* tan t'ien.

hatha yoga   A mostly physical system of yoga; literally sun-moon union. It encompasses postures, breathing, and mental discipline.

hoch'mah   The Hebrew word for a divine energy related to intuitive wisdom.

hoku   Large intestine 4, a powerful acupuncture point that affects the large intestine as well as the nervous system. When properly stimulated, hoku can be used to produce anesthesia during major surgery, and is also excellent for treating headaches.

hologram   A 3-D image produced by wave interference patterns and stored on a 2-D surface.

holographic access system   The author's designation for a system of energy healing where a clearly defined part of the body can be used as a map to diagnose and/or treat the entire energy matrix. Examples of such systems in use are the feet, hands, ears, face, irises, etc.

homeopathy   A healing modality created by Samuel Heinemann in the late eighteenth century. Homeopathic remedies are prescribed based upon their ability to mimic the disease state in a healthy individual, thereby stimulating the sick body to heal itself.

huna   A Hawaiian word meaning "secret," the esoteric wisdom of Polynesia and the energy healing system native to it.

hypothalamus   A mid-brain center that regulates and connects the autonomic nervous system with the glandular system; houses the centers for satiety, hunger, and sleep and produces the beta-endorphins that are the body's natural painkillers.

hz   *See* cps.

iconoclast   An idol smasher, someone who tries to break up outdated ideas and dogmas he or she believes are no longer valid and build new visions of the world.

iridiagnosis/iridology   The holographic access system of the eye, used for diagnosis in energy healing.

Kabbalah   The Jewish mystical tradition and its teachings.

kapha   One of three major metabolic types in Ayurvedic medicine.

karma   The Sanskrit word for action; refers to the ledger of good and bad deeds that stay with a person through one life and into the next.

kavana   A Hebrew word that means directed consciousness, attention, intention, or disciplined spiritual imagination.

khamsin   Positive ion wind storms that plague the Middle East and affect the electrical charge of the body's cells.

ki   A Japanese term for life force energy.

Kirlian photography   A form of high-voltage photography that photographs light around animate and inanimate objects not visible to the naked eye.

kundalini   The serpent energy that rises through the chakras and liberates the consciousness of the yogi.

kung fu   Literally, hard work and practice or discipline. It often, but doesn't necessarily have to, refers to a martial arts system.

L-fields   A term created by Dr. Harold Saxton Burr to refer to the controlling, organizing electrical life fields of the living form; an electrical matrix that molds living matter.

limbic system   The part of the brain that controls autonomic functions.

macrobiotics   A diet-oriented natural healing system focused on keeping the yin/yang polarity of the energy matrix in balance by eating certain foods in a certain way.

mal'ach   The Hebrew word for angel or messenger.

mana   A Hawaiian word for the life-force energy, according to the huna system.

mantra   A syllable or sound vibration to help focus the mind during meditation or prayer.

meridians   Channels of energy in Chinese medicine that run throughout the body, which carry chi.

mesmerism   A term used for the hypnotic trance state in the early days of hypnosis, named after Dr. Franz Anton Mesmer.

mikvah   The Jewish ritual bath used for purification, containing water from a living source (rain, springs, lakes, rivers, oceans, etc.).

monopoles   Sub-atomic particles that are so small they have only one electrical pole, such as an electron.

moxa   The Chinese word for the mugwort herb; when burning, its heat is used to stimulate acupuncture points.

moxibustion   A Chinese medicine technique for stimulating acupuncture points with heat generated by holding a burning stick of moxa (mugwort) near an acupuncture point, or burning a small clump of the herb at the end of an acupuncture needle.

nadis   In yoga, energy channels that carry needed prana/energy around the energy matrix; the energy equivalent of the body's nervous system.

naturopathy   A system of alternative medicine based on the principle of vitalism, which focuses on natural self-healing based on lifestyle changes.

neh'fesh   One of the Hebrew words for the soul, from the root "to breathe."

Newtonian physics   Classical physics, dealing with the physical world of the senses: what can be seen, heard, smelled, tasted, and touched.

nih'shah'mah   One of the Hebrew words for the soul, from the root "to breathe."

Ohr Ayn-Sof   In Hebrew, literally, "Light of the Infinite"; refers to the slower dimensions of God's light that human beings can experience; *See* Ayn-Sof.

Olam   A Hebrew word for world; in Kabbalah, it refers to the four worlds or dimensions of the universe: the physical, emotional, mental, and spiritual; olamot (p).

orgone   Life-force energy, according to Wilhelm Reich.

osteopathy   A system of manual therapy that relies on knowledge of the structure (anatomy) and function (physiology) of the body to treat diseases, disorders, and dysfunctions.

paradigm   Worldview; a set of ideas that guide a person's life.

parasympathetic nervous system   The part of the autonomic nervous system that evokes the relaxation response after a stressful event triggers the fight-or-flight response.

phase-lock   In the context of energy healing, this is what occurs when the brain waves of one individual entrains with another so that their energy matrices are "talking" to each other.

pitta   One of the three major metabolic types in Ayurvedic medicine.

pituitary gland   The master endocrine gland of the body.

placebo   A harmless and ineffective substitute (usually a sugar pill) for the real medication in laboratory research; a way of testing the efficacy of a new drug or treatment.

prana   The Sanskrit word for the life-force energy according to yoga.

psychometry   The ability to pick up vibrations and information about an object's history, ownership, etc., simply by touching it.

qi   *See* chi.

Qi Gung   *See* Chi Gung.

quantum physics   The branch of physics that deals with the principles and behavior of the very small and super-large aspects of matter and energy, such as atoms and subatomic particles.

quarks   Subatomic particles inside the proton of an atom.

RB (Reflex Balance)   The author's holographic access system of foot and hand massage that emphasizes anatomical accuracy of its charts, incorporates breathing and rooting into its protocol, and chakras and meridians into its model.

reflexology   A healing modality of foot or hand massage; one of many holographic access systems in use around the world.

relaxation response   The mechanism that relaxes the body after a stressful situation has passed.

Reiki   A Japanese term for the life force; a system of energy healing utilizing the flow of Reiki energy.

Ru'ah   One of the Hebrew words for the soul, meaning spirit, wind, or breath.

rhythmic entrainment   When the frequency of an individual or object vibrates at the same frequency as another individual or object, they are said to be phase-locked or in rhythmic entrainment.

scalar fields   Extremely low frequency magnetic fields; the fingers that push the DNA keyboard buttons in a patient.

scalar waves   *See* E.L.F. or scalar fields.

sefer yetzirah   *The Book of Creation*, one of the oldest and most mysterious of all Kabbalistic texts.

sefirah   In Kabbalah, the Hebrew word for the building block energies of the universe; the 10 divine intelligences that are the foundation of creation; sefirot (p).

shiatsu   The Japanese system for finger-pressure massage of the body.

Sufism   The mystical branch of Islam.

sushumna   In yoga, the central spine of the energy matrix along which the energy of the subtle body reside and through which the kundalini rises.

sympathetic nervous system   The branch of the autonomic nervous system that evokes the fight-or-flight response.

t'ai chi   Literally, supreme ultimate, representing the balance of forces within the universe, the two halves of which are the yin and the yang. An internal Chinese martial arts exercise system.

t'ai chi ch'uan   An internal Chinese martial arts exercise system.

t'ai chi t'u   An expansive Chinese diagram that shows how the energy and physical universes are related. The yin/yang circle diagram is sometimes referred to by the same designation.

tan t'ien   The body's lower center of gravity, 2 or 3 inches below and behind the navel; the core energy focal point for breathing, martial arts, and deep meditative practices.

teh chi   Literally, "obtaining the energy"; in acupuncture, a slight electric shock during treatment which indicates that a needle has made contact with a meridian.

theta   The brain wave designation for a very deep, relaxed state, in the range of 4–7 hz.

Torah   The Five Books of Moses; used as a general term for the entire Jewish Bible.

Tree of Life   The visual representation of the Kabbalistic *sefirot*.

triasphere   Along with the two known physical hemispheres of the brain, this is the author's designation for a third, non-physical receiving part of the energy mind.

vata   One of the three major metabolic types in Ayurvedic medicine.

WEB   The worldwide energy bubble; the infinite ocean of energy that encompasses the entire universe.

wu shu   Literally, martial arts; a relatively modern term, usually referring to the more vigorous styles of various kung fu empty-handed and weapons systems.

yantra   A geometric design used as a focal point in meditation.

yin/yang   The two complementary forces of the universe that, working together, maintain its equilibrium. The "double-fish" diagram symbolizing the duality of the universe.

yoga   The union of body, energy, and spirit, an ancient and diverse system of philosophy and practice for achieving a heightened state of awareness and improving health.

zhen jui   The Chinese name for acupuncture, literally meaning needle heat.

Resources

Websites

The author's website contains all of the instructional videos mentioned in the text, on breathing, rooting, ocular divergence, massage, and scanning.

www.andronenergyhealing.org

National Center for Complementary and Alternative Medicine

http://nccam.nih.gov/

Natural Solutions Magazine, www.naturalsolutionsmag.com

Acupuncture

American Association of Acupuncture and Oriental Medicine www.aaaomonline.org/

American Academy of Medical Acupuncture www.medicalacupuncture.org

Energy Medicine

The International Center for Reiki Training, www.Reiki.org

Therapeutic Touch: Classes and information can be obtained by contacting Pumpkin Hollow Retreat Center (www.pumpkinhollow.org) or Therapeutic Touch International Associates, the official organization of Therapeutic Touch (www.therapeutic-touch.org).

Homeopathy

National Center for Homeopathy

www.homeopathic.org

Music

www.StevenHalpern.com. Healing music, free samples, videos, and articles on his breakthrough perspectives on sound healing, subtle energies, and supporting our physical and spiritual health and well-being.

Nutritional Medicine

American Association of Naturopathic Physicians, www.naturopathic.org

Books

Benson, Herbert, M.D. with Klipper Miriam Z. *The Relaxation Response.* New York: HarperCollins Publishers Inc., 2004.

Brennan, Barbara Ann, *Hands of Light: A Guide To Healing Through The Human Energy Field.* New York: Pleiade Books, 1987.

Emoto, Masaru, D.A.M. *The Hidden Messages in Water.* Hillsboro, OR: Beyond Words Publishing, Inc., 2004.

Kaplan, Aryeh, Rabbi. *Inner Space.* Brooklyn, NY: Moznaim Publishing Corporation, 1990.

Kaptchuk, Ted J., O.M.D. *The Web That Has No Weaver: Understanding Chinese Medicine.* New York: Contemporary Books, A Division of McGraw Hill, 2000.

Kreiger, Dolores, Ph.D., R.N. *The Therapeutic Touch: How to Use Your Hands to Help or to Heal.* Englewood Cliffs, NJ: Prentice-Hall Inc., 1979.

Lockie, Andrew, M.D. *Family Guide to Homeopathy: Symptoms and Natural Solutions.* New York: Fireside Press, A Division of Simon and Shuster, 1993.

Mann, Felix, M.B. *Acupuncture: The Ancient Chinese Art of Healing and How It Works Scientifically*. New York: Random House, 1972.

Motoyama, Hiroshi, M.D. with Brown, Rande. *Science and the Evolution of Consciousness: Chakras, Ki and Psi*. Brookline, MA: Autumn Press, 1978.

Puharich, Andrijah, M.D. *Beyond Telepathy*. New York: Doubleday, 1962.

Rossi, Ernest L. Ph.D. *The Psychobiology of Mind-Body Healing: New Concepts of Therapeutic Hypnosis*. New York: W.W. Norton & Company, Inc., 1986.

Trivieri, Jr., Larry and Anderson, John W., Editors. *Alternative Medicine: The Definitive Guide*. New York: Celestial Arts, A Division of Random House, 2002.

Index

T

U–V

W

X–Y–Z